MENSTRUATION,
HEALTH,
AND ILLNESS

SERIES IN HEALTH CARE FOR WOMEN
Series Editor: **Phyllis Noerager Stern**, DNS, RN, FAAN

Helpers in Childbirth: Midwifery Today   Oakley and Houd
Silent Sisters: An Ethnography of Homeless Women   Russell
Menstruation, Health, and Illness   Taylor and Woods

In Preparation

*Violence Against Women: Nursing Research, Education,
    and Practice Issues*   Sampselle

MENSTRUATION, HEALTH, AND ILLNESS

Edited by

Diana L. Taylor
*Women's Health Program
and Family Health Care Nursing
School of Nursing
University of California
San Francisco, California*

Nancy F. Woods
*Parent and Child Nursing
and Center for Women's Health Research
University of Seattle
Seattle, Washington*

●HEMISPHERE PUBLISHING CORPORATION
A member of the Taylor & Francis Group

New York   Washington   Philadelphia   London

MENSTRUATION, HEALTH, AND ILLNESS

1 2 3 4 5 6 7 8 9 0   B R B R   9 8 7 6 5 4 3 2 1

This book was set in Times Roman by Hemisphere Publishing Corporation. The editors were Nancy Niemann, S. Michele Nix, and Carolyn V. Ormes. Production manager was Peggy M. Rote; typesetters were Laurie Strickland and Deborah S. Hamblen. Cover design by Debra Eubanks Riffe. Printing and binding by Braun-Brumfield, Inc.

A CIP catalog record for this book is available from the British Library.

Library of Congress Cataloging-in-Publication Data

Menstruation, health, and illness / edited by Diana L. Taylor, Nancy F. Woods
        p.   cm.—(Series in health care for women)
    Based on papers presented at the seventh conference of the Society
for Menstrual Cycle Research, held at the University of Mich. in Ann
Arbor in June 1987.
    Includes bibliographical references and index.

    1. Premenstrual syndrome—Congresses.   2. Menstruation—
Congresses.   3. Menopause—Congresses.   4. Women—Psychology—
Congresses.   I. Taylor, Diana L.   II. Woods, Nancy Fugate.
III. Society for Menstrual Cycle Research.   IV. Series.
    [DNLM: 1. Menstrual Cycle—congresses.   2. Premenstrual Syndrome—
congresses.   3. Women—Psychology—Congresses.   WP 540 M54 87 1987]
RG165.M46   1991
618.1'72—dc20
DNLM/DLC
for Library of Congress   91-7005
                                                                                CIP

ISBN 1-56032-132-6
ISSN 1047-4005

Contents

Contributors

Connie Gleim Bareford, RN, MA, PhD
Associate Professor, Department of
  Nursing
William Paterson College of New
  Jersey
Wayne, NJ 07470, USA

Carole Bartz, MSW
The Phoenix Clinic, Inc.
2421 N. Mayfair Road, Suite 200
Wauwatosa, WI 53226, USA

Erik J. Bergstralh, MS
Section of Biostatistics
Mayo Clinic and Mayo Foundation
Rochester, MN 55905, USA

Daniel J. Cardona, MD
Department of Psychiatry
University of Michigan
1500 E. Medical Center Drive
Ann Arbor, MI 48109-0120, USA

Joan C. Chrisler, PhD
Assistant Professor, Department of
  Psychology
Connecticut College
New London, CT 06320, USA

C. James Chuong, MD
Division of Reproductive
  Endocrinology and Infertility
Department of Obstetrics and
  Gynecology

Smith Tower, 8th Floor
6550 Fannin
Houston, TX 77030, USA

Robert C. Colligan, PhD
Head, Section of Psychology
Mayo Clinic and Mayo Foundation
and Professor of Psychology
Mayo Medical School
Rochester, MN 55905, USA

Linda L. Coughlin, RNC, MBS
Nurse Practitioner, Obstetrics and
    Gynecology
Mountain View Ob/Gyn
3910 Carefree Circle South, Suite B
Colorado Springs, CO 80917, USA

Carolyn B. Coulam, MD
Consultant, Department of Obstetrics
    and Gynecology
Mayo Clinic and Mayo Foundation
and Professor of Obstetrics and
    Gynecology
Mayo Medical School
Rochester, MN 55905, USA

Lolafaye Coyne, PhD
Research Department, Menninger
Box 829
Topeka, KS 66601-0829, USA

Barbara Shelden Czerwinski, RN, MSN
Assistant Professor, School of Nursing
University of Texas Health Science
    Center
1100 Holcombe Blvd.
Houston, TX 77030, USA

Denys deCatanzaro, PhD
Department of Psychology
McMaster University
Hamilton, Ontario L8S 4K1, CANADA

Greer Glazer, RN, PhD
Associate Professor, Parent Child
    Nursing Graduate Program,
School of Nursing, Kent State
    University
Kent, OH 44242-0001, USA

John F. Greden, MD
Professor and Chair
Department of Psychiatry
University of Michigan,
1500 E. Medical Center Drive
Ann Arbor, MI 48109-0120, USA

Elizabeth E. Guice, PhD
1022 Bedford Road
Grosse Pointe Park, MI 48230
and Adjunct Professor, Institute of
    Gerontology
Wayne State University
Detroit, MI 48202

Eleni G. Hapidou, PhD
Research Associate, Lecturer,
    Department of Psychology
Social Science Center
University of Western Ontario
London, Ontario N6A 5C2, CANADA

Roger F. Haskett, MD
Director, Depression Program
Department of Psychiatry
University of Michigan
1500 E. Medical Center Drive
Ann Arbor, MI 48109-0120, USA

Cynthia Hedricks, PhD
Assistant Professor, Department of
    Occupational Therapy
University of Southern California
2250 Alcazar St., CSA-203
Los Angeles, CA 90033, USA

Donna S. Huddleston, RN, PhD
Research Specialist
Room 1126, College of Nursing

845 S. Damen, M/C 802
University of Illinois
Chicago, IL 60612, USA

Janice J. Jurgens, RNC, MS
Clinician, Planned Parenthood of
    Rochester and the Genesee Valley
Rochester, NY 14607
and Adjunct Instructor, School of
    Nursing
University of Rochester
Rochester, NY 14642, USA

Kathryn A. Lee, RN, PhD
Assistant Professor, Family Health Care
    Nursing, N411Y
University of California
San Francisco, CA 94143-0606, USA

Martha J. Lentz, RN, PhD
Research Assistant Professor,
    Physiological Nursing, SM-23
University of Washington
Seattle, WA 98195, USA

Beverly J. McElmurry, EdD, FAAN
Professor
Room 1120, College of Nursing
845 S. Damen, M/C 802
University of Illinois
Chicago, IL 60612, USA

Peg Miota, BSN, ACSW
Director of Outpatient and Community
    Services Center
Milwaukee Psychiatric Hospital
1220 Dewey Ave.
Wauwatosa, WI 53213, USA

Ellen S. Mitchell, ARNP, PhD
Research Assistant Professor, Parent
    and Child Nursing, SM-23
University of Washington
Seattle, WA 98195, USA

Julene Morgan, BS
Senior Research Assistant, The Tremin
    Trust Research Program
College of Nursing, Room 501
University of Utah
Salt Lake City, UT 84112, USA

John W. Phillis, PhD, DSc, DVSc
Professor and Chair, Department of
    Physiology
Gordon H. Scott Hall of Basic Medical
    Sciences
School of Medicine
Wayne State University
540 E. Canfield Ave.
Detroit, MI 48201, USA

Linda J. Piccinino, MPS(ID)
Carolina Population Center
University of North Carolina
Chapel Hill, NC 27516-3997, USA

Bethel A. Powers, RN, PhD
Associate Professor of Nursing and
    Education
University of Rochester School of
    Nursing and Graduate School of
    Education and Human Development
Rochester, NY 14642, USA

Margie Ripper, PhD
Research Fellow, Women's Studies
Flinders University of South Australia
Bedford Park, South Australia 5042,
    AUSTRALIA

Mary Ellen Robertson, MSN, ARNP
Florida Atlantic University
1834 NE 34th St.
Fort Lauderdale, FL 33306, USA

Janet Root, MSN, PhC
Data Manager, The Tremin Trust
    Research Program
and Project Director, MRH Follow-Up
    Study
College of Nursing, Room 501

University of Utah,
Salt Lake City, UT 84112, USA

Alice Sutton Rozman, ND, RN
2562 Princeton Rd.
Cleveland Heights, OH 44118, USA

Joseph Sargent, MD
Headache and Internal Medicine
    Research Center, Menninger
Box 829
Topeka, KS 66601-0829, USA

Ken R. Smith, PhD
Associate Professor and Associate
    Director, The Tremin Trust Research
    Program
and Department of Family and
    Consumer Studies
University of Utah
Salt Lake City, UT 84112, USA

Patricia Solbach, PhD
Headache and Internal Medicine
    Research Center, Menninger
Box 829
Topeka, KS 66601-0829, USA

Rajiv Tandon, MD
Director, Schizophrenia Program
Department of Psychiatry
University of Michigan
1500 E. Medical Center Drive
Ann Arbor, MI 48109-0120, USA

Diana L. Taylor, RN, PhD
Director, Women's Health Program
and Assistant Professor, Department of
    Family Health Care Nursing
School of Nursing, Room N411-Y, Box
    0606
University of California
San Francisco, CA 94143-0606, USA

J. Richard Udry, PhD
Carolina Population Center
University of North Carolina
Chapel Hill, NC 27516-3997, USA

Ann M. Voda, RN, PhD
Professor and Director, Tremin Trust
Research Program
College of Nursing, Room 501
University of Utah
Salt Lake City, UT 84112, USA

Nancy F. Woods, RN, PhD, FAAN
Professor, Parent and Child Nursing
and Director, Center For Women's
    Health Research, SM-23
University of Washington
Seattle, WA 98195, USA

Mary Yahle, RN, CS, MSN
Outpatient and Community Service
    Center
Milwaukee Psychiatric Hospital
1220 Dewey Ave.
Wauwatosa, WI 53213, USA

Preface

The seventh conference of the Society for Menstrual Cycle Research, held at the University of Michigan in Ann Arbor in June 1987, continued the work of previous meetings to provide a forum for research and knowledge about menstrual cycle phenomena. Founded in 1978, The Society for Menstrual Cycle Research is an organization of scientists, scholars, clinicians, students, and consumers who share an interest in women's lives and health needs as these relate to the menstrual cycle. The theme for the seventh conference focused on sexual influences on the menstrual cycle and was titled "Sexuality and the Menstrual Cycle: Clinical and Sociocultural Implications." Dr. Winifred Cutler provided the keynote address, which focused on the role of the menstrual cycle in sexual behavior of women.

In addition to the main theme, the seventh conference focused on (a) psychosocial, cultural, and historical aspects of the menstrual cycle, (b) theoretical issues and management considerations for premenstrual syndrome, and (c) future directions in menstrual cycle research. Dr. Roger Haskett provided a keynote address introducing the methodologic dilemmas of perimenstrual symptom research. Representing the increasingly broad interdisciplinary focus of these conferences, Tambrands Corporation supported the first annual lectureship for the Society. Dr. Barbara Czerwinski spoke on future directions in menstrual cycle research in her provocative and unusual presentation titled "Feminine Hygiene and Space." In addition to the keynote presentations, approximately 50 papers were presented to an international audience of 150 attendees.

In order to include as many presentations as possible in this publication, we solicited all of the papers presented at the seventh conference. While some were published elsewhere, 20 papers are included and were updated. In a number of papers the data were reanalyzed, and the contemporary findings are included here. The papers represent a sampling of the interdisciplinary work presented at the seventh conference. We have organized the papers into sections. Part One focuses on the experience of menstruation from neuroendocrinological and sociocultural perspectives. Part Two focuses on the theoretical and clinical aspects of perimenstrual symptoms and syndromes. Part Three is a collection of papers that explore the normative and illness orientation of research and knowledge related to menopause.

We hope that this collection of papers provides the reader with the intellectual excitement and professional stimulation that this conference provided the authors and audience in Ann Arbor in 1987. The Society for Menstrual Cycle Research conferences have been catalysts for new and innovative thinking in the area of the menstrual cycle. Subsequent conferences will continue this work: in 1989, the Society held its eighth conference at the University of Utah in Salt Lake City, and in June 1991 it held the ninth conference at the University of Washington in Seattle.

The convener for the seventh conference was Dr. Nancy Reame from the University of Michigan, who is Vice President of the Society for Menstrual Cycle Research. Also important to the success of the conference and this publication were the officers and board of directors of the Society: Dr. Judith Abplanalp, President; Dr. Barbara Sommer, Second Vice President and Newsletter Editor; Dr. Mary Anna Friederich, Secretary/Treasurer; Dr. Alice Dan; Dr. Sharon Golub; Dr. Michelle Harrison; Dr. Linda Lewis; Dr. Jerilynn Prior; Dr. Kathleen Ulman; and Esther Rome. We thank all of them for their support, guidance, and leadership in the development of the Society for Menstrual Cycle Research, the organization of the seventh conference, and the finalization of this publication.

Diana L. Taylor
Nancy F. Woods

Part One

The Experience of Menstruation

At menarche, women are forced to adapt to neurohormonal cyclicity involving the hypothalamic-pituitary-adrenal-ovarian system. For 30–40 years after the onset of menarche women experience the rise and fall associated with ovarian hormones and subsequent interaction with other neurohormonal events. The cyclicity of menstruation has a profound effect on women's lives. Not only a physiological process, menstruation is associated with feminine role development and feelings of health and well-being, and it is embedded in the sociocultural context of women's experience.

The papers reported in this section contribute to the knowledge of the experience of menstruation; an experience that encompasses psychosocial, cultural, neuroendocrine, and technological dimensions. Voda, Morgan, Root, and Smith (Chapter 1) report on the Tremin Trust, an intergenerational research program and database for studying the events associated with women's menstrual and reproductive lives. This research program and database, initiated in 1934, resides at the University of Utah and currently includes 1,316 active intergenerational and crosscultural recordkeepers. The Tremin Trust is the largest active database providing prospective information on events associated with women's menstrual and reproductive lives.

In a prospective study of the comparative impact of the "social cycle" and menstrual cycle on Australian women's mood performance and sexual interest, Ripper (Chapter 2) found that mood was affected by both menstrual and social cycle. The statistical analyses provide a strong illustration of the social mediation of the menstrual cycle. Ripper suggests that women filter their mood and sexual sensations through competing interpretive frameworks: perception of menstrual cycle phase and weekend or weekday. She defines these interpretive frameworks as "cognitive constructs," which operate at a background, subliminal level for the individual woman.

Little is known about the beliefs about menstruation in American cultural subgroups. Jurgens and Powers (Chapter 3), in an exploratory study of Headstart mothers, studied their menstrual euphemisms, beliefs, and taboos. These data provide important baseline information about a particular ethnic culture of women, and the authors also provide reflections on the implications for research, education, and clinical practice.

Improved technology allows us to study the interactive effects of the neuroendocrine environment in relation to the menstrual cycle. Cardona, Tandon, Haskett, and Greden (Chapter 4) review the evidence for alterations in the activity of various neurotransmitter and endocrine systems across the menstrual cycle and present data indicating that hypothalamic-pituitary-adrenal function varies with the phase of the menstrual cycle. In studying serum cortisol after a dexamethasone suppression test in women diagnosed with major depression, these authors suggest that the menstrual cycle must be considered in the interpretation of results of various neuroendocrine tests.

Phillis (Chapter 5) reports on research focused on the effects of the menstrual cycle at intracellular and neuronal level. This author reviews the research-based literature on the effects of steroid hormones on hypothalamic-pituitary-adrenal neuron activity related to adenosine. He reports data suggesting that modifications of adenosinergic inhibitory tone, resulting in enhanced (17β-estradiol) or reduced (progesterone) neuronal excitability may represent important elements of the communication between the body and the brain that is essential for appropriate integrated behavioral response. Phillis applies this knowledge to clinical therapeutics, suggesting that manipulation of adenosinergic substances (caffeine, theophylline, methylxanthines) may provide a convenient and accessible route for the control of these imbalances.

In another study of the relationship between behavior and the neuroendocrine events associated with the menstrual cycle, Hedricks, Piccinino, and Udry (Chapter 6) ask two questions: Do changes in women's hormones at midcycle affect coital behavior? And, can menstrual cycle length estimate the luteinizing hormone (LH) surge onset day? Since biological specimens with which to determine LH surge onset day are not available to all investigators, the authors attempted to estimate LH surge onset day using a nonhormonal measure (menstrual cycle length). Although there was a strong positive correlation between cycle length and LH surge onset day, cycle length alone was not sufficient to accurately predict LH surge onset day. The estimation did not yield the observed midcycle peak in coitus on LH surge onset day. However, LH surge onset day at midcycle appears to be a biologically meaningful reference point from which to explore changes in human behavior across the menstrual cycle.

Chapter 7 provides an interesting and futuristic look at the experience of menstruation. Czerwinski, a consultant to the NASA Space Station Personal Hygiene Study, discusses the research related to Earth practices for the personal hygiene activity of feminine hygiene in space. This author describes space travel in the future that will involve large numbers of people living and working together for long periods of time under confined conditions in a hostile environment. Czerwinski poses research questions and ideas to guide hygiene procedures related to the menstrual cycle and space travel.

Chrisler, in Chapter 8, the final chapter in Part One, investigates changes in creative thinking across the menstrual cycle in regularly menstruating healthy women and compares them to a control group of men. Although no significant differences in cognitive function were found for women during premenstruum, one third of the women perceived their performance to be impaired during the premenstrual phase.

Chapter 1

The Tremin Trust:
An Intergenerational Research Program on Events Associated with Women's Menstrual and Reproductive Lives

Ann M. Voda, Julene Morgan, Janet Root, and Ken R. Smith

INTRODUCTION

The Tremin Trust Research Program on Women's Health was initiated in 1934 under the directorship of Dr. Alan E. Treloar at the University of Minnesota. The project, initially called the Menstruation and Reproductive History (MRH) program, was designed to collect data prospectively on events associated with women's menstrual and reproductive lives. The original goal of the research was to determine the magnitude of the variability in the menstrual experience among women.

Contrary to evidence available at that time, Treloar (1979) suggested that "regularity" as applied to the menstrual cycle was a vague term and should not be taken literally to mean without variation. Instead, according to Treloar, the "cycle" needed to be reconceptualized as a complex variable. Treloar also postulated that there was no such thing as an average cycle and that duration of bleeds and intervals between bleeds differed from one woman to another as well as varying from one cycle to another within the same woman. Thus, the need for a large number of individual menstrual histories, each covering several years of experience, became apparent. Commencing in 1935, a large group of university women was recruited for the sole purpose of recording onset and stop of menstrual bleeds. Treloar hoped that sufficient data could be gathered to disprove the common myth that women menstruated regularly, every 28 days. Since its inception, however, the scope of the program has been expanded.

In January of 1984, after Dr. Treloar's retirement, the program was acquired by the University of Utah College of Nursing. Dr. Ann M. Voda was appointed program director. The Trust, at present, is a nonprofit research program supported largely through grant awards and contributions. It is the only ongoing program of its kind in the world.

PARTICIPANTS

Three primary groups of women were enrolled in the MRH program between 1934 and 1965.

Group 1: 1930s Panel

Women enrolled at the University of Minnesota volunteered to be participants in the study between 1934 and 1939. Initially, a pilot group of 525 women were recruited through physical education classes and sororities. Another 1,825 women were enrolled through the Student Health Center. Because health examinations were required of all students when entering the university, during this procedure each woman was given information about the study and invited to participate. These two groups of women comprised the original panel.

Group 2: 1960s Panel

Three decades later, between 1961 and 1963, to facilitate a comprehensive analysis of the variation in the menstrual cycle over time, a new student panel comparable to the original one was recruited. This time, however, enrollment of participants was done through the mail, because the health examinations were performed by the students' family physicians. This recruitment effort resulted in the enrollment of 1,367 women.

Group 3: Alaskan Panel

In 1965, the MRH program was expanded to include a panel of 1,000 Alaskan women and girls to provide data on whether or not seasonal variations, such as the widely varying length of the solar day, influenced the menstrual cycle. At that time, the assistance of the Arctic Health Research Center was requested to recruit participants and to collect data on menstruation and reproduction. All menstruating Eskimo, Aleut, and native Indian women residing in nine rural villages located in the Yukon-Kuskokwim delta region of southwestern Alaska were invited to participate in the study. Later, native women in two larger commercial centers, Bethel and Barrow, were enrolled to augment the village women.

After the MRH program was established in the native villages, 170 Caucasian women in urban environments in Alaska were also enrolled. The purpose of enrolling the Caucasian women was to isolate the effects of seasonal variations from those of heredity and lifestyle. Though this panel was small, Treloar (1979) believed that the numbers were adequate. To date, 51 of the 170 Alaskan Caucasian women remain in the study. No native women have continued as recordkeepers.

Group 4: Intergenerational Participants

One of the main features of the MRH, renamed the Tremin Trust in 1984 is the intergenerational nature of the data. In 1946 daughters of the first group, the 1935–1939 panel, reached menarche and were enrolled as participants. In mid-1972, granddaughters of the original panel were enrolled. Currently, daughters and granddaughters from both groups have been (and continue to be) enrolled in the study. There are 836 mother-daughter pairs and 72 mother-daughter-granddaughter sets in the database. Of these women, 313 mother-daughter pairs and 22 mother-daughter-granddaughter sets are active. These figures were accurate as of 1986. There is great potential to study trends and effects through the intergenerational file.

Current Active Participants

At present, approximately 1,316 women representative of all four groups previously described, age range early teens to mid-90s, are enrolled in the project as active recordkeepers. Of the 1,316 active participants, 852 are menstruating and 464 are nonmenstruating. The Trust participants have a proven commitment to the project. The return rate on the 1987 health report survey mailed to more than 1,500 women was 75%. After the mailing list was updated and women lost to the project were eliminated, the return rate on the 1988 health report form was 87%.

The age distribution of active participants is bimodal, heavily weighted toward the enrollment periods of groups 1 and 2 with daughters, granddaughters, and Alaskan women filling in between and to the right and left of those two peaks. The age distribution of all active participants is shown in Figures 1-1 and 1-2.

The original participants of The Trust were enrolled when they were students at the University of Minnesota and this has influenced the demographics. Specifically, the majority of women are of Scandinavian descent and college educated. At present, 41% of all active participants continue to reside in Minnesota. The remaining 59% reside in the other states and some foreign countries. Residence sites and number of participants in each site are shown in Figure 1-3.

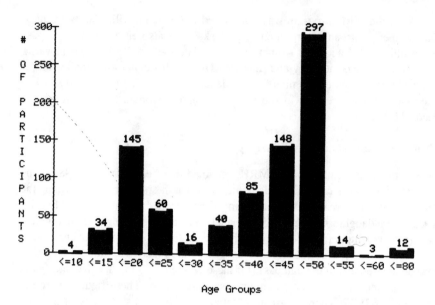

Figure 1-1   Age distribution of active menstruating participants as of 12/31/88.

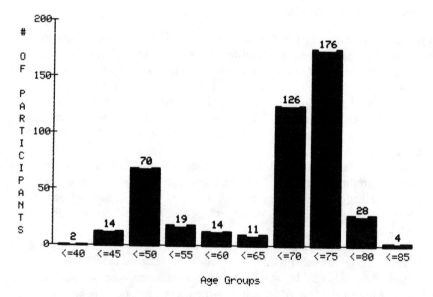

Figure 1-2   Age distribution of active nonmenstruating participants as of 12/31/88.

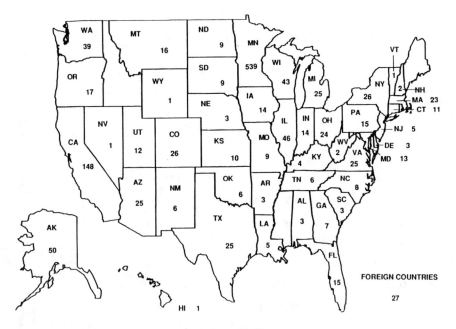

Figure 1-3 Distribution of active participants, 1989.

DATA COLLECTION INSTRUMENTS

Three primary instruments have been used to collect data: a menstrual calendar card, a medical report form, and, commencing in 1987, a health report form. In addition, over the years, special surveys have been done to study various topics. Over the past 55 years, many women have volunteered interesting anecdotes about menstruation, menopause, birthing, and, for some, the records contain information that reveals the unfolding of lives from adolescence to old age. None of the volunteered information has been analyzed.

Menstrual Calendar Card

The emphasis of the research program has been on the prospective collection of menstrual data and this continues to be a primary focus. The menstrual cycle card shown in Figure 1-4 was designed by Treloar (1979) and has been used to gather data on menstruation start and stop since the program's inception in 1934. The card consists of consecutive dates through the year arranged in lines of 28 days each. According to Treloar, consecutive circled dates on this grid would reveal instantly, by a straight line formation in vertical and transverse array, the degree of regular menstrual periodicity. Any departure from this formation was considered "irregular." In addition, duration of the menstruation would likewise become evident for its extent and variability in the horizontal grouping of dates. The reverse of the card was designed to provide space for entry of anecdotal informa-

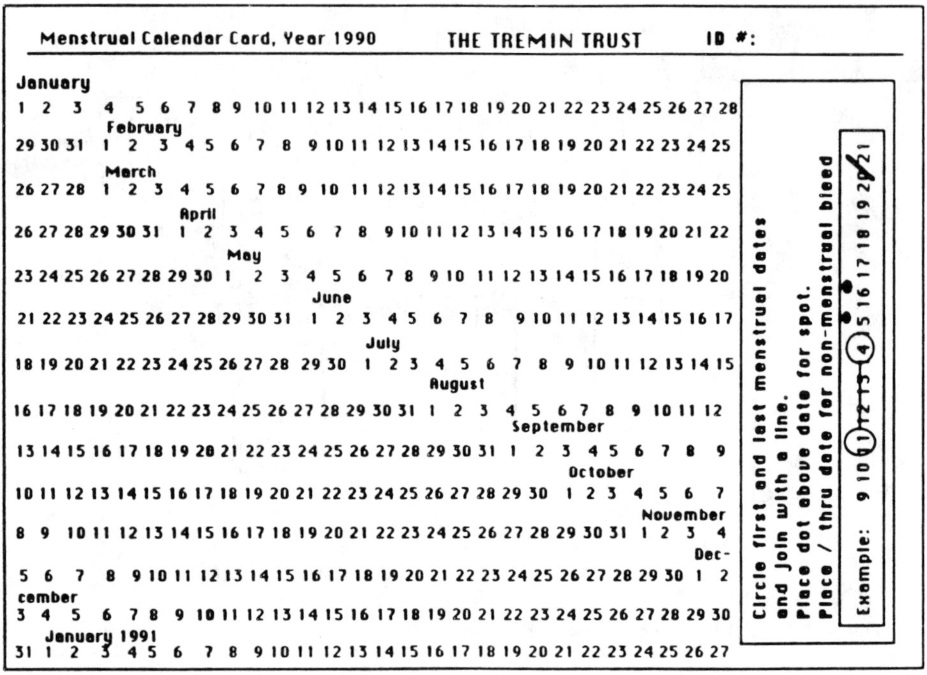

Figure 1-4   Menstrual calendar card, front.

tion concerning events that were perceived to affect the menstrual experience. In January of each year, menstrual calendar cards are mailed to participants as part of the annual mailing. At the year's end, completed cards are returned with the health report form for the same year. The card, developed by Treloar, has proven to be extremely useful as a research instrument. To the best of our knowledge The Trust is the only study wherein the dates of both menarche and menopause are collected. The date of menopause is documented prospectively by the participants. Because the majority of the daughters of participating women are invited to join the study just before the onset of their menstruation, the date of menarche is frequently captured as it happens.

Annual/Medical Report Form

In 1935, largely for administrative purposes, a 1-page annual report form was implemented to obtain information on marital status, occupation, and any medical treatments participants had had during the previous year for menstrual difficulties. Thus, in contrast to the prospective nature of menstruation data obtained via the menstrual calendar card, the annual report form was designed to gather data retrospectively. The form was modified through the years to meet requests for specific information and the expanding medical objectives of the program. Records of past pregnancies and live births were added in 1937 to obtain information on reproductive histories. In 1952, when members of group 1 were approaching menopause, information on menopause was included. At this time, information to determine whether or not daughters of group 1 who were approaching menarche might be interested in joining the study was also included. Commencing in 1963, information on oral contraceptive usage, surgeries other than those on the reproductive system, and the occurrence of accidents and other stressful life events was included. In 1965, the annual report form was renamed the "medical report form." At this time, information about initiation of oral contraceptives was requested. Intrauterine device (IUD) usage and other contraceptive measures were added in 1971. In 1974 sex and weight

Please make notations here of:
(1) Any flow period for which an accurate record was omitted from the calendar for any reason. This is VERY IMPORTANT
(2) Any events which you think might have altered your normal menstrual pattern or which caused you to bleed between periods. This includes records of surgery (named), illnesses, medications, or any life event.
(3) An explanation of any symbols you may have used on the other side of this card.

The Tremin Trust
Menstrual Calendar Card for 1990
This is a research Document
University of Utah College of Nursing

Figure 1-4   Menstrual calendar card (*Continued*), back.

of births and abortion information were requested. In 1975 information on tubal ligations, breastfeeding, and whether or not a husband/partner had had a vasectomy was requested. In 1977 the final addition to the medical report form occurred, wherein information on malignant cancer was requested. A typical 1-page medical report form is shown in Figure 1-5.

Health Report Form

In 1987 the medical report form was expanded to a 5-page "health report form" as the need to focus more broadly and holistically on women's health became apparent. As Treloar so aptly stated, the menstrual cycle is "a life within a life" (Treloar, 1979). Before 1987 no information had been systematically obtained to determine how socioeconomic and behavioral factors might interact with biological factors to affect the health of women over the life course. Hence, the 1-page form was expanded to begin to meet this objective. Questions on living arrangements, income levels, caregiving and receiving, exercise, infertility, the personal meanings of menstruation and menopause, and smoking histories were included.

At present, in January of each year a health report form and a new menstrual calendar card are mailed to menstruating participants, and a health report form is sent to nonmenstruating participants. All participants complete and return the health report form, giving their health status during the previous year. Menstruating women return the completed menstrual calendar card from the previous year with the health report form. The new menstrual calendar card is retained to be filled out during the current year.

Special Surveys

In addition to completing monthly calendar cards and yearly reports, some select groups of women have participated in special surveys. Thus, requests for special information applicable to a relatively small number of women were no longer included in the general medical report. Such requests were included in special surveys and were mailed only to those women who had experienced the event in question and who had indicated a willingness to respond. Examples of special surveys conducted utilizing Trust participants are (1) Special Health Report on Mammary Health; (2) Special Report on Family Relationships; (3) Special Report on Surgery for Blocking or Opening the Fallopian Tubes; (4) Special Health Report on the Relationships of Breast Cancer, Uterine Surgery, and Smoking History; (5) Special Report on Oral Contraceptive Usage and Possible Side Effects; (6) Special Health Report on Diseases or Conditions of the Reproductive System, Other Special Conditions, or Diseases; (7) Report on Diethylstilbestrol (DES) usage; (8) Mother-Daughter Relationships in Menopause and the Aging Process; and (9) Special Women's Health Survey, which examines the connection between lifelong menstrual patterns and a variety of health outcomes.

MRH RESEARCH PROGRAM : 1986 MEDICAL REPORT

NAME: _____   Tel.: (_____)_____-_____   Card # _____
changed(   )

ADDRESS: _____
changed(   )   street   city   state   zip-code
                                      MARITAL STATUS changed in 1986 to: S   M
                                                                           W   D   Sep.

PLEASE REPORT ON EACH ITEM BELOW (1986 only)

1. 1986 CALENDAR CARD is ENCLOSED(   ), or LOST(   ).   (Please use ✓ or X in appropriate box(   )).

2. CARD has been rechecked carefully to make sure that any OMISSION has been NOTED(   ).

3. PREGNANCY in '86 NO(   ). Or YES(   ): CONTINUES into '87(   ), or was TERMINATED on ___/___ by LIVE BIRTH(   ),
   mo. day

   or STILLBIRTH(   ), or INDUCED ABORTION(   ), or SPONTANEOUS MISCARRIAGE(   ). LATTER was SUSPECTED(   ), or

   CONFIRMED by LABORATORY(   ), or by DOCTOR(   ).

4. PREGNANCY CONTROLS: NO(   ). or YES(   ):

   (a) OC PILLS were CONTINUED(   ), or STARTED on ___/___, or STOPPED on ___/___, &/or CHANGED(   ) on ___/___
                                         mo. day   mo. day   mo. day

       to _____. REASON: _____→
          name & strength   FOR START, STOP OR CHANGE

   (b) An IUD was CONTINUED(   ), or REPLACED on ___/___, or INSERTED(   ) on ___/___, &/or WITHDRAWN(   ) on
                                       mo. day   mo. day

       ___/___. TYPE used:_____. REASON _____→
       mo. day   for action taken

   (c) TUBAL SURGERY(   ), or PARTNER"S SURGERY(   ) on ___/___.
                                                       mo. day

   (d) Other procedure: DIAPHRAM CONDOM FOAM RHYTHM or _____→
                                                       please specify

5. HORMONES used for non-contraceptive purposes: ESTOGENS THRYROID CORTISONE INSULIN or _____→
                                                                                  please specify

   use was CONTINUED(   ), or STARTED(   ) on ___/___, &/or STOPPED on ___/___.
                                           mo. day   mo. day

6. MENOPAUSE is CONFIRMED (no bleeding all year)(   ), or is suspected(   ) because _____→

7. HYSTERECTOMY: NO(   ). Or YES(   ), on ___/___. Reason:_____→
                                         mo. day

8. Other SURGERY: NO(   ). Or YES(   ), on ___/___. Please specify_____→
                                          mo. day

9. MALIGNANCY diagnosed: NO(   ). Or Yes(   ), on ___/___ Please specify _____→
                                                 mo. day

10. ACCIDENT or STRESS: NO(   ). Or Yes(   ), on ___/___ Please specify _____→
                                                mo. day

11. HOSPITAL INPATIENT: NO(   ). Or YES(   ), from ___/___ to ___/___ for _____→
                                                  mo. day   mo. day   please specify

12. My DAUGHTER is interested in the MRH program . NAME: _____ AGE: ____

    Pre-menarche(   ) or MENARCHE on ___/___/___. Please send materials to me(   ) (or to her(   )).
                                    mo. day yr.

NOTES or COMMENTS _____

_____

_____

_____

→ Please continue on other side of page, or by item number on another sheet if necessary.

Figure 1-5 Medical report form used from 1977 to 1986.

DATA

The Trust's archival database is computerized and approximately 170 mega-bytes in size with well over 1.2 million computer records. Coincident with the development and use of computers in research, creation of protocols to govern coding operations of menstrual and report form data commenced in 1965. At present, the computerized database is stored on a Micro VAX operated by The University of Utah School of Medicine, Clinical Research Center Computer Center.

Coded Data

In the late 1960s, data stored in manila files were transferred to magnetic tape to formulate a master file. Types of events coded since the 1960s and the cumulative frequencies of occurrence of each event coded on the master file for calendar years 1935 to 1980 are displayed in Figure 1-6.

Of the 2,350 women who were enrolled in the 1930s, 240 have contributed 30 years of data. On average, each of these 240 participants had contributed more than 21 years of data as of 1980. The average number of "missing" years of data for this same group, years in which no data were reported, is very low, 2.75 years. The number of years of participation in the research program for the 1,316 active participants is shown in Figure 1-7.

RESULTS

In 1967 the first article resulting from analyses of recorded menstruation start and stop records kept by group 1 was published (Treloar, Boynton, Borghild, & Brown, 1967). This article described the variability in menstrual interval in women across the life span. Since 1967, many research articles have been published utilizing data obtained via the menstrual calendar card, annual/medical report forms, and special surveys. The published research findings have generated information on the following topics: gestational interval (Treloar, Borghild, & Cowan, 1967; Behn & Treloar, 1968; Hammes & Treloar, 1970); effects of breastfeeding on postpartum menstruation, ovulation, and pregnancy in Alaskan natives (Hellman, Berman, & Hanson, 1972); menarche, menopause, and intervening fecundability (Treloar, 1974); effects of oral con-traceptives on the human menstrual cycle (Treloar & Behn, 1974; Taylor, Berger, & Treloar, 1977; Berger, Taylor, & Treloar, 1977); variation in the human menstrual cycle (Treloar, 1974, 1981); secular trend in age at menarche (Treloar, Boynton, & Cowan, 1974); estimation of the parameters of a type I geometric distribution from truncated observations on conception delays (Das Gupta & Hickman, 1974); effects of ignoring dropout cases on fecundability (Das Gupta & Hickman, 1976); seasonal behavior of human menstrual cycle (Sundararaj, Chern, Gatewood, Hickman, & McHugh, 1978; Albright, Voda, Smolensky, Hsi, & Decker, 1990); menstrual cycle patterns and breast cancer

EVENT CODE	DESCRIPTION	FREQ.	EVENT CODE	DESCRIPTION	FREQ.
00	1st day of menses	528715	51	chronic illness diagnosed	199
01	1st day after menses	515656	52	stress w/o treatment	1267
02	ovulation sign	1153	53	non-trivial bodily injury	122
03	1st day of spotting	20547	54	genital bleeding, post-meno	72
04	1st day after spotting	20451	55	menstrual disorder ceases	40
05	1st day non-menst bleed	2217	56	mental/stress w/treatment	119
06	1st day after non-menst bleed	2183	57	hospital admit-nonsurgery	114
07	1st day of unknown bleed	661	58	hospital discharge-nonsurgery	110
08	1st day after unknown bleed	652	59	special interest condition	262
09	menarche	3962	60	sequential OC starts	291
10	1st marriage recorded	1959	61	progestin-only OC starts	4
11	1 hormone tx, for menst dis	244	62	100+ mg estrogen OC starts	839
12	1 hormone tx, other dis	41	63	75-80 mg estrogen OC starts	280
13	1 or 1st urogen x-ray tx	26	64	50-60 mg estrogen OC starts	714
14	1 or 1st non-urogen x-ray tx	32	65	35 mg or less estrogen OC starts	54
15	1 or 1st non-surgery tx	823	66	IUD inserted	506
16	horm tx, sustained, menst dis	2140	67	IUD removed, no reaction	225
17	1st day post code 16	223	68	other method BC starts	1706
18	horm tx, sustained non-menst	283	69	other method BC stops	390
19	1st day post code 18	84	70	fertility hormone starts	153
20	unassigned code	1	71	unassigned code	0
21	1st live birth	1639	72	hormone tx for meno starts	254
22	2nd live birth	1295	73	hormone tx for meno stops	137
23	3rd live birth	657	74	unknown OC starts	847
24	4th live birth	280	75	OC use terminated	2943
25	5th live birth	114	76	IUD reaction, no action taken	66
26	6th live birth	46	77	IUD reaction, removal	183
27	7th live birth	20	78	BC reaction, no action taken	1
28	8th live birth	8	79	BC reaction, use terminated	2
29	9th live birth or more	8	80	unassigned code	0
30	stillbirth	30	81	unassigned code	2
31	spont abortion-confirmed	653	82	death	35
32	spont abortion-unconfirmed	163	83	withdraw, non-medical reason	165
33	ectopic preg, term by surgery	20	84	withdraw, medical reason	3
34	induced abortion	72	85	menses stop, self-reported	5
35	breastfeeding starts	1205	86	menses stop, post x-ray tx	13
36	1st day post breastfeeding	1090	87	menses stop, post hormone tx	2
37	synthetic feeding starts	121	88	menses stop, post OC use	1
38	no mention of feeding method	400	89	break in history	8024
39	vasectomy of partner	122	90	menopause confirmed	295
40	D and C	739	91	menopause w/spotting	6
41	sterilization	248	92	menopause inferred	165
42	hysterectomy	279	93	terminated by director	5
43	oophorectomy, 1st unilateral	62	94	meno confounded w/horm tx	90
44	oophorectomy, bilateral	17	95	natural amenorrhea	1
45	urogen procedures	572	96	amenorrhea, x-ray induced	0
46	abdom/rectal surg	301	97	amenorrhea, other tx induced	0
47	other surgery	303	98	amenorrhea, post OC use	2
48	urogen surgery	136	99	contact lost	1673
49	unspecified surgery	32		ABBREVIATIONS: tx= treatment,	
50	menstrual/genital disorder	1506		OC= oral contraceptive, BC= birth control	

Figure 1-6 Cumulative frequency of event codes, 1934–1980.

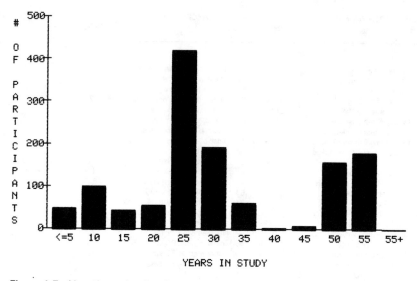

Figure 1-7   Years in study of active participants through 1980.

risk factors (Wallace, Sherman, Bean, Leeper, & Treloar, 1978); variations in the reporting of menstrual histories (Bean, Leeper, Wallace, Sherman, & Treloar, 1979); spontaneous abortion (Wilcox, Treloar, & Sandler, 1981; Wilcox & Horney, 1984; Wilcox & Gladen, 1982; Wilcox, 1983); age at menarche and subsequent reproductive events (Sandler, Wilcox, & Horney, 1984); probability of menopause with increasing duration of amenorrhea in middle-aged women (Wallace, Sherman, Bean, Treloar, & Schlabaugh, 1979); risk of post-pill amenorrhea (Berger, Taylor, & Treloar, 1977); predicting the end of menstrual life (Treloar, 1982); effect of menstrual and reproductive factors on age at menopause (Whelan, Sandler, McConnaughey, & Weinberg, 1990); and the mother-daughter relationship in menopause and the aging process (Patsdaughter, in press; Patsdaughter & Killean, 1990).

ACCESSING THE TREMIN TRUST RESEARCH PROGRAM

Qualified researchers and other interested individuals or organizations can request information on how to access the database and/or the participants. The procedure is to submit a brief, yet clear proposal in the form of a letter to The Trust. The proposal should include a statement of the problem, specific research questions, how accessing The Trust data or participants will facilitate answering the research questions, and methodology that will be employed to analyze or collect data. After initial review by The Trust staff, the proposal will be either returned for more information or forwarded to The Tremin Trust Advisory Committee for review.

REFERENCES

Albright, D. L., Voda, A. M., Smolensky, M. H., Hsi, B. P., & Decker, M. (1990). Seasonal characteristics of and age at menarche. In *Chronobiology: Its Role in Clinical Medicine, General Biology, and Agriculture, Part A* (pp. 709-720). New York: Wiley-Liss.

Albright, D. L., Voda, A. M., Smolensky, M. H., Hsi, B. P., & Decker, M. (in press). Seasonal characteristics of and age at menarche. *Chronobiology International.*

Bean, J. A., Leeper, J. D., Wallace, R. B., Sherman, B. M., & Treloar, A. E. (1979). Variation in the reporting of menstrual histories. *American Journal of Epidemiology, 109,* 181-185.

Behn, B. G., & Treloar, A. E. (1968). Gestational interval from general hospital and private practice records. *Biology of the Neonatal, 12,* 363-370.

Berger Jr., G. S., Taylor, R. N., & Treloar, A. E. (1977). The risk of post-pill amenorrhea: A preliminary report from the Menstrual and Reproduction History Research Program. *International Journal of Gynaecological Obstetrics, 15,* 125-127.

Das Gupta, O., & Hickman, L. (1974). Estimation of the parameters of a type I geometric distribution from truncated observation on conception delays. *Mathematical Biosciences, 22,* 75-78.

Das Gupta, O., & Hickman, L. (1976). A note on the effect of ignoring dropout cases on fecundability as estimated from a follow-up study. *Journal of Theoretical Biology, 61,* 411-417.

Hammes, L. M., & Treloar, A. E. (1970). Gestational interval from vital records. *American Journal of Public Health, 60,* 1496-1505.

Hellman, I. L., Berman, M. L., & Hanson, K. (1972). Effect of breastfeeding on postpartum menstruation, ovulation, and pregnancy in Alaskan Eskimos. *American Journal of Obstetrics and Gynecology, 144,* 524-534.

Patsdaughter, C. (in press). Mother and daughter in menopause and the aging process: Empirical models and nursing implications. *Monograph: Second Annual Helen T. Milian Lectureship in Nursing Research Conference.*

Patsdaughter, C., & Killean, M. (1990). Developmental transitions in later life: Mother-daughter relationship. *Holistic Nursing Practice, 4*(3), 37-46.

Sandler, D. P., Wilcox, A. J., & Horney, L. F. (1984). Age at menarche and subsequent reproductive events. *American Journal of Epidemiology, 119*(5), 765-774.

Sundararaj, N., Chern, M. M., Gatewood, L. C., Hickman, L., & McHugh, R. (1978). Seasonal behavior of human menstrual cycles: A biometric investigation. *Human Biology, 50,* 15-31.

Taylor, R. N., Berger Jr., G. S., & Treloar, A. E. (1977). Changes in menstrual cycle length and regularity after use of oral contraceptives. *International Journal of Gynaecological Obstetrics, 15,* 55-59.

Treloar, A. E. (1974). Menarche, menopause and intervening fecundability. *Human Biology, 46,* 89-107.

Treloar, A. E. (1976). Variation in the human menstrual cycle. *Proceedings of the Research Conference on National Family Planning,* (pp. 64-71). Washington, D.C.: Human Life Foundation.

Treloar, A. E. (1979). Menstruation and Reproduction: Historical review of a research program, 1934-1979 (unpublished manuscript).

Treloar, A. E. (1981). Menstrual cyclicity and the pre-menopause. *Maturitas, 3,* 249-264.

Treloar, A. E. (1982). Predicting the end of menstrual life. In A. Voda, et al. *Changing perspectives on menopause.* Austin: University of Texas Press.

Treloar, A. E., & Behn, B. G. (1974). Effect of oral contraceptives on the menstrual cycle. *Proceedings of the Fourth World Congress on Fertility and Sterility* (pp. 886–890). Tokyo and Kyoto, Japan, Netherlands: Excerpta Medica.

Treloar, A. E., Borghild, B. G., & Cowan, D. W. (1967). Analysis of gestational interval. *American Journal of Obstetrics and Gynecology, 99*(1), 35–45.

Treloar, A. E., Boynton, R. E., Borghild, G. B., & Brown, B. W. (1967). Variation of the human menstrual cycle through reproductive life. *International Journal of Fertility, 12*(1), 77–126.

Treloar, A. E., Boynton, R. E., & Cowan, D. W. (1974). Secular trend in age at menarche, U.S.A.: 1893–1974. *Proceedings of the Eighth World Congress on Fertility and Sterility* (pp. 25–28). Buenos Aires, Argentina, Netherlands: Excerpta Medica.

Wallace, R. B., Sherman, B. M., Bean, J. A., Leeper, J. P., & Treloar, A. E. (1978). Menstrual cycle patterns and breast cancer risk factors. *Cancer Research, 38,* 4021–4024.

Wallace, R. B., Sherman, B. M., Bean, J. A., Treloar, A. E., & Schlabaugh, L. (1979). Probability of menopause with increasing duration of amenorrhea in middle-aged women. *American Journal of Obstetrics and Gynecology, 135,* 1021–1024.

Whelan, E. A., Sandler, D. P., McConnaughey, D. R., & Weinberg, C. R. (1990). Menstrual and reproductive characteristics and age at natural menopause. *American Journal of Epidemiology, 135*(4), 625–632.

Wilcox, A. J. (1983). Surveillance of pregnancy loss in human populations. *American Journal of Industrial Medicine, 4,* 285–291. Also in Mattison, D. R. (ed.): *Reproductive Toxicology.* New York: Alan R. Liss Co.

Wilcox, A. J., & Gladen, B. C. (1982). Spontaneous abortion: The role of heterogeneous risk and selective fertility. *Early Human Development, 7,* 165–178.

Wilcox, A. J., & Horney, L. F. (1984). Accuracy of spontaneous abortion recall. *American Journal of Epidemiology, 120*(5), 727–733.

Wilcox, A. J., Treloar, A. E., & Sandler, D. P. (1981). Spontaneous abortion over time: Comparing occurrence in two cohorts of women a generation apart. *American Journal of Epidemiology, 114*(4), 548–553.

Chapter 2

A Comparison of the Effect of the Menstrual Cycle and the Social Week on Mood, Sexual Interest, and Self-Assessed Performance

Margie Ripper

INTRODUCTION

Throughout the past 60 years there has developed a belief, supported by a great deal of research, that all women experience some degree of menstrual cycle variation in mood, performance, and sexual interest. The most common explanation for this reporting of cyclical change is that hormonal levels (and/or related biochemical factors) determine the variation. So it is that our society has come to see hormones as a major determinant of women's competence, ability, stability, and rationality. A further aspect of this contemporary view of the menstrual cycle is that the low points in cyclical variation have come to be seen as dysfunctions or medical disorders to which all menstruating women are potentially susceptible. Thus menstrual cycle variation has become synonymous with illness categories.

A systematic study of the empirical evidence on which this view of the menstrual cycle is based shows that the findings are confusing and often contradictory, and in many cases "facts" about the menstrual cycle are created by the research's instruments and design. Shortcomings in the orthodox menstrual cycle research have been highlighted in a number of methodological critiques undertaken in the past decade (Laws, 1983; Gannon, 1981; Ruble & Brooks-Gunn, 1979; Parlee, 1982). The present study draws on and extends these critical analyses. In particular, this study challenges the dominant assumption that menstrual cycle variations are negative and constitute illness or disability. The study also provides a comparative perspective on the strength of the menstrual cycle effect on women's lives by making a simultaneous comparison of the menstrual cycle with that of the social cycle (whether it is weekend or a weekday).

This study is important because it adds to the methodological sophistication of menstrual cycle research and challenges the assumption that diseases and disorders are fixed or "given" entities that can be investigated objectively. Instead, they are produced through a social process that includes the negotiation of their definition, their etological explanations, and the way in which they are experienced by those people identified as suffering from them. Researchers and clinicians are active participants in the process through which diseases and disorders are developed. The emergence of menstrual cycle research is grounded in the sociopolitical context of medicine within Western industrialized countries. Consequently, it reflects developments within that context, including changes in the medico/scientific understanding of reproduction. It mirrors the conflict and confusion produced by the competing knowledge offered by different professional interest groups. It is a response to technological and marketing influences. Ultimately, it has become a central focus in debates about women's roles and rights. The present study demonstrates that these broader concerns have influenced what is researched and, consequently, what is currently believed about the menstrual cycle. There are several ways in which orthodox menstrual cycle research has embedded stereotypical beliefs about women into the design of the studies and thereby reproduced those stereotypes as facts in the results. This author will identify only those areas of concern that have direct relevance to the design and the interpretation of this study.

A major assumption embedded within the measurement instruments is that the menstrual cycle produces negative effects. In many instruments the only (or predominant) factors being measured are negative ones. For example, the widely used Moos Menstrual Distress Questionnaire contains 47 items, 43 of which are negative (Moos, 1985).

Much research focuses only on those phases of the study presumed to be problematic (predominantly the premenstrual and menstrual phases) to the exclusion of the remainder of the cycle. This focus reproduces the a priori assumption that these phases are characterized by illness or dysfunction.

Retrospective self-report questionnaires are widely used despite having been shown to reproduce cultural stereotypes about menstrual cycle experience rather than providing a valid measure of a particular woman's experience (Parlee, 1974; Ruble & Brooks-Gunn, 1979; Englander-Golden, Whitmore & Dienstbier, 1978).

The problem of selection bias plagues existing research and limits the generalizability of results. Although menstrual cycle effects are presumed to exist to varying extents in all menstruating women, much of the research has been carried out with women from narrow, nonrepresentative subgroups of the population. Many study samples are drawn from hospital/clinical or university populations. The generalizability to findings to "women at large" is questionable. The focus on nonrepresentative subgroups of women prevents the systematic investigations of sociodemographic characteristics such as age, socioeconomic or employment status, ethnicity, fecundity, or contraceptive usage. This omission means that hormonal/biochemical factors are separated from the context of women's lives. This separation results in a reinforcement of a reductionist biological (hormonal) etiology of the menstrual cycle as it prevents the simultaneous study of biological and sociocultural factors and the possible interaction between them.

Studies that rely on volunteer samples (such as PMS sufferers) are likely to select from one extreme of the spectrum of the women's menstrual cycle experience. These studies also accentuated the demand effect, which has been shown to operate if participants are aware that the study is focusing on the menstrual cycle (Englander-Golden, Sonleitener, Whitmore, & Carbley, 1986). Several critical studies have shown the tendency for cultural stereotypical experience to be reported in studies where women's attention had been focused on the menstrual cycle (Koeske & Koeske, 1979; Parlee, 1982). There are now such well-established expectations attached to the menstrual and premenstrual phases of the cycle that there is an increased likelihood that negative symptomology and events will be attributed to the menstrual cycle rather than to external factors. In studies where the participants are aware that the research focus is on the menstrual cycle this attribution is accentuated (Englander-Golden et al., 1986).

Very few studies are able to provide comparative measures against which the strength (and practical significance) of menstrual cycle changes can be compared. Thus there is no possibility of placing the effect of the menstrual cycle in perspective alongside other physiological and life events that are known to influence mood and performance. For example, the circadian rhythm in body temperature or the fluctuations in blood sugar levels across the day are both physiological cycles that influence our sense of well-being *possibly* in greater amplitude than does the menstrual cycle. One example of a social cycle is the effect of the social week (i.e., the way our lives and activities vary from weekend to weekday). Other events and activities in our lives also have an impact on mood and performance (e.g., the amount of caffeine or alcohol consumed or the amount of sleep or exercise may have a greater impact on our sense of well-being than does the menstrual cycle). The lack of comparative perspective on the practical impact of the menstrual cycle on women's lives sustains the belief that it is a major limitation to which all women potentially succumb. The present study provides a comparison of the effect of the menstrual cycle with the social week. The study also identifies the pattern of menstrual cycle change in normal woman who prospectively record their mood, sexual interest, and self-assessed performance using an instrument that allows equal opportunity to record positive and negative experiences.

METHODS

Recruitment of Participants

Women from an urban South Australian community participated in a study of the menstrual cycle in which they were required to record daily self-report questionnaires for a minimum of 5 weeks, or for as long as they were willing to do so. The participants were recruited by the researcher from a variety of nonclinical situations such as social and sporting clubs, women's groups, school, mothers' clubs, and adult education classes. Each participant completed a prestudy questionnaire that provided demographic data and details of health, menstrual cycle, and contraceptive experience. An analysis of this information showed the sample to be quite representative of the adult, urban-dwelling, South Australian population of women from which it was drawn. The median age of participants was 31–35 years (thus the study is not generalized to adolescent women or to older women approaching or having reached menopause). Somewhat fewer of the participants had children (60%) than in the South Australian population in general, where 67% of women of equivalent age are mothers. A slightly higher rate of employment was evident in the study sample than in the equivalent population. Of the participants, 70% were employed at least on a part-time basis (30% worked in the home or were unemployed), whereas 64% of South Australian women of equivalent age are employed (Australian Bureau of Statistics, 1981). On the basis of the pre-study questionnaire, 43% of the participants reported experiencing premenstrual symptoms that were of concern to them. This is a lower rate than would be expected from survey research. However, it is notoriously difficult to judge the incidence and to compare reports of such a loosely defined disorder as PMS. Problems with menstruation were reported by 39% of the sample. This rate is consistent with the incidence of menstrual pain reported by Wood, Larsen, & Williams (1979) in a similar population. Although the sample was not randomly selected, it is reasonably reflective of adult Anglo South Australian women.

The following analysis reports the experience of 55 of the participants who were not taking oral contraceptives, had not reached menopause, had not undergone a hysterectomy, and were not pregnant or lactating. These women are categorized as "ovulating" women and were selected for this analysis because they are likely to represent the range of normal menstrual cycle experience. Validation of ovulation was not possible without increasing the focus and salience of the menstrual cycle and ovulation in particular. However, a subgroup of 10 of the women participated in an additional study, where they undertook physiological monitoring, in addition to the daily questionnaires, throughout one further menstrual cycle. The physiological monitoring involved continuously recorded deep body temperature using a Vitalog physiological recorder. Also, urine was analyzed using the pregnanediol test. These data allowed the thermal shift and the progesterone rise to be identified, thus establishing the existence and timing of ovulation. In all 10 cases, these more reliable measures confirmed that ovulation had occurred, thus lending support to the categorization of the 45 similar women as "ovulating." The Vitalog study also confirmed the accuracy of McIntosh, Matthews, Crocker, Broom, & Cox (1980) technique for calculating the timing of ovulation based on overall cycle length. This technique was utilized in the designation of the "ovulation phase" of each woman's cycle.

The Questionnaire

A daily self-report questionnaire was designed using polar opposite adjective scales to allow equal likelihood of positive and negative experiences being reported. Removal of the negative bias from the measurement instrument ensured that positive menstrual cycle variation (if such a thing existed) could become evident. This technique is a departure from traditional menstrual cycle research, where instruments list only (or predominantly) negative symptoms (Moos, 1968; Taylor, 1979) and have women report the extent to which they occur. In addition to these polar opposite scales, the daily questionnaire sought information on sleep length and quality, physical sensations and symptoms, life events, and consumption of stimulants and medication. Thus a comprehensive study of the menstrual cycle in the context of a woman's life is possible from these data. This paper reports only on the measures of mood performance and sexual interest. Twelve scales were developed (Table 2-1), eight of which cover the feelings and emotions most commonly reported as being cyclically influenced. Three scales were developed to measure self-perceived performance, and a single scale was included to measure sexual interest. Table 2-1 provides a list of the 12 polar opposite adjective scales with the descriptors underlined that reflect the negative symptoms of which conventional menstrual cycle questionnaires are typically comprised.

Phasing of the Cycle

To include the entire cycle and to allow comparison of equivalent points in cycles in different lengths, the following five phases were distinguished, defining the first day of the cycle as the day on which menstrual bleeding began. The five phases were constructed as:

Table 2-1   Polar Opposite Scales on Which Daily Moods Were Recorded

How Did You Feel Today? (Place one tick (√) in the appropriate position on each of the scales below.)

	In between	
Relaxed	: ____ : ____ : ____ : ____ : ____	: Tense
Irritable	: ____ : ____ : ____ : ____ : ____	: Calm
Dominant	: ____ : ____ : ____ : ____ : ____	: Submissive
Light hearted	: ____ : ____ : ____ : ____ : ____	: Depressed
Bungling	: ____ : ____ : ____ : ____ : ____	: Competent
Stable	: ____ : ____ : ____ : ____ : ____	: Moody
Trusting	: ____ : ____ : ____ : ____ : ____	: Suspicious
[a]Lethargic	: ____ : ____ : ____ : ____ : ____	: Energetic
[a]Withdrawn	: ____ : ____ : ____ : ____ : ____	: Sociable
Creative	: ____ : ____ : ____ : ____ : ____	: Unimaginative
Confident	: ____ : ____ : ____ : ____ : ____	: Vulnerable
[b]Randy	: ____ : ____ : ____ : ____ : ____	: Disinterested in sex

[a]Measures of performance.
[b]Pilot studies showed that this Australian euphemism was the adjective that most reliably described feeling sexually interested.

Menstrual phase: All days of menstrual bleeding. (This phase varied in length from individual to individual and from cycle to cycle.)

Premenstrual phase: Seven days before the onset of menstrual bleeding.

Ovulation phase: A 3-day phase comprising the day on which ovulation was calculated most probably to have occurred, plus 1 day preceding and 1 day following that day. The ovulation day was calculated (retrospectively) on the basis of the length of that cycle, using the formula developed by McIntosh et al. (1980) and validated in 10 of the participants through the urine analysis and Vitalog core temperature recording described previously.

Preovulation phase: Included all days following the menstrual phase and preceding the ovulation phase; thus this phase varied in length.

Luteal phase: Included all days following the ovulation phase and before the premenstrual phase, again a phase of variable length.

On the basis of this categorization every daily questionnaire for an individual woman was allocated to a particular phase of the cycle. The SPSSX aggregate program sorted each daily questionnaire according to whether it was recorded on a weekend or a weekday *and* according to the phase of the cycle to which it belonged. For each woman, a mean score on each of the polar opposite scales was calculated for each phase of the cycle for weekend and weekday data separately. This allowed each woman's data to be weighted equally in the analysis regardless of the number of days of data collection and regardless of differences in cycle lengths. The data matrix produced by the aggregate program allowed a doubly repeated MANOVA analysis to be made for the group as a whole. From these analyses the following research questions were investigated:

1   Does the menstrual cycle have a negative effect on a normal woman's mood performance and sexual interest?

2   What is the comparative impact of the social cycle and menstrual cycle on a woman's mood performance and sexual interest?

3   Do the social cycle and menstrual cycle interact to affect a woman's mood?

The inclusion of the entirely socially constructed variable social cycle allows a comparison to be made between the impact of a woman's menstrual cycle with the impact of the social context. This comparison provides a perspective on how "disabling" the menstrual cycle is compared with the "disabling" effect (to which both women and men are subject) of it being a weekday rather than a weekend. If the menstrual cycle pattern is the same, regardless of whether it was a weekday or weekend, then the social cycle would appear to be less consequential in influencing women compared with the impact of the menstrual cycle. If on the other hand, the social and menstrual cycles interact or if the social cycle (weekend effect) was equally as strong an influence on women's mood as was the menstrual cycle, then the dominant belief that the menstrual cycle is a major influence on women would be difficult to sustain.

RESULTS

Positive and Negative Effects of the Menstrual Cycle

The first important finding of this study concerns the overwhelmingly positive rather than negative picture of menstrual experience, which emerges when the research instrument allows equal likelihood of positive and negative moods being reported. On each of the 5-point polar opposite scales, the midpoint was 3; scores above 3 therefore indicated positive emotions rather than negative. For the group as a whole, none of the measures of mood or performance fell below the midpoint at any time during the menstrual cycle. Only the measure of sexual interest was reported as negative; women felt uninterested in sex in both the premenstrual and menstrual phases.

It can be concluded that in this study there is no premenstrual or menstrual mood change of sufficient intensity to be felt as tension, irritability, depression, moodiness, suspiciousness, vulnerability, or feelings of submission or unimagination. The women did not report themselves to be lethargic, bungling, or withdrawn.

The menstrual cycle did have an impact on most of the moods and perceptions of performance; however, it is more accurate to describe this variation as positive, rather than as negative. The MANOVA repeated measures analysis showed that all of the measures, except for feelings of dominance and trust, changed significantly ($f \leq .01$) across the menstrual cycle. Figure 2-1 graphs

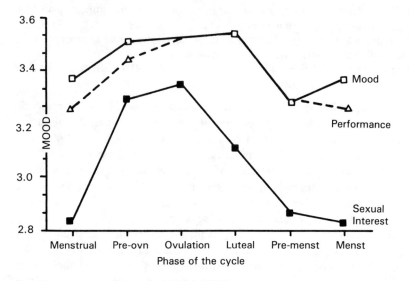

Figure 2-1 Comparison of the pattern of variation across the menstrual cycle of mood, performance, and sexual interest. Mood includes feeling relaxed, calm, lighthearted, stable, creative, and confident. Performance includes feeling competent, energetic, and sociable. Mean scores for the group as a whole ($N = 55$).

the pattern of change in mood, performance, and sexual interest reported by the women across five phases of the cycle. (The menstrual phase is plotted both at the left and right of the graph to allow easier comparison with the premenstrual phase.) Figure 2-1 represents the average score that the group of women reported in each phase of the cycle for each of the three dimensions (i.e., mood, performance, and sexual interest).

It is clear from Figure 2-1 that the average mood and performance for the women does fluctuate depending on phase of the menstrual cycle. However, it remained positive (above the midpoint of the scale) at all times. Women's sexual interest varied more dramatically than did other feelings and reached the negative level both premenstrually and during menstruation.

Figure 2-1 indicates that women felt less positive in the premenstrual and menstrual phases than during the phases surrounding and including ovulation. This menstrual cycle effect would better be described as Great Ovulation Elation Syndrome (GOES) than PMS or menstrual cycle-related depression, dysfunction, or dysphoria. The importance of this observation is not, however, to create yet another syndrome but to illustrate the power that measurement instruments have in creating data. The overwhelming tendency in menstrual cycle research has been to seek measures only (or predominantly) of negative symptoms. The Moos Menstrual Distress Questionnaire (Moos, 1969) epitomizes this tendency, and the recently developed diagnostic criteria for late luteal phase dysphoric disorder (LLPDD) reproduces this tradition (DSMP-III-R, 1987). The use of polar opposite scales demonstrates that when negative bias is removed a quite different picture of menstrual cycle variation emerges; one that is incompatible with the common belief that the menstrual cycle has a negative effect on women's lives. This finding challenges the belief that PMS and menstrual dysphoria are ubiquitous. It also reinforces that the methodological problems discussed previously are not merely examples of sloppy research design. Rather, they are examples of the way in which dominant beliefs about the menstrual cycle and women's inherent "illness" are embedded within and thus reproduced through research.

The Effect of the Social Context on Women's Menstrual Cycle and Well-Being

Australian society is structured around a strict delineation of weekend from weekday. Weekends are a time for relaxation, time away from work, and time for family and/or leisure activities. Even for those women with domestic responsibilities, weekends are characteristically less routine and less driven by external constraints than are weekdays. Given this strong ideology of enjoyment, one would expect that many of the measures of mood and physical well-being would be more positive on the weekend than during the week. The analysis showed that on 4 of the 12 moods the social week had a main effect—that is, the women felt consistently more relaxed ($f = .000$), calm ($f = .001$), trusting ($f = .024$), and sexually randy ($f = .048$) when it was a weekend than they did on weekdays, regardless of phase of their menstrual cycle. Conversely, women felt more dominant during the week than they did on weekends ($f = .023$). This quite unremarkable finding that one's mood can be affected by the social environment has been documented elsewhere (Rossi & Rossi, 1988); however, it is worth emphasizing that, although this social cycle exists and is associated with lower weekday moods, this is not *experienced* as weekday tension, irritability, suspicion, and sexual disinterest. Equivalent variation in moods across the menstrual cycle, however, does carry negative connotations and implies an illness label for which all women are eligible. Table 2-2 provides a comparison of the effect of the menstrual and social cycles of each of the measures mood, performance, and sexual interest.

In addition to the main differences between weekday and weekend feelings, there was some evidence that the social week mediates the way in which women experience their menstrual cycle. For example, the cyclic pattern of sociability across the cycle was significantly different ($f = .04$) when it was a weekend than on weekdays. Stated differently, the impact of the weekend on women's sociability differed depending on the phase of the cycle. Figure 2-2 shows the differing cyclical pattern between weekend and weekday. The pattern shows that menstruation, premenstruation, and luteal phases are experienced similarly

Table 2-2   List of Variables with Level of Significance of Main Effect and Interaction Effect for Each

Variable	Main effect of phase f	Main effect of social week f	Interaction between phase and social week f
Moods			
Relaxed/tense	.000	.000	—
Calm/irritable	.000	.001	—
Dominant/submissive	—	.023	—
Lighthearted/depressed	.000	—	—
Stable/moody	.001	—	—
Trusting/suspicious	—	.024	—
Creative/unimaginative	.012	—	—
Confident/vulnerable	.000	—	—
Performance			
Competent/bungling	.000	—	—
Energetic/lethargic	.000	—	—
Sociable/withdrawn	.000	—	.036
Sexual interest			
Randy/disinterested in sex	.000	.048	—

whether it is a weekday or weekend. The ovulation phase is dramatically different, with women feeling much less sociable when they ovulate on a weekend rather than when they do so on a weekday. Conversely, the preovulation phase is associated with increased sociability when it coincides with the weekend.

This pattern is echoed consistently on all of the other mood and performance variables (but not on sexuality); however, the interaction effect does not reach a level of statistical significance ($f \leq .05$) on any of the other variables (Table 2-2). Despite the statistical weakness of the interaction of each measure when analyzed separately, there is a remarkable consistency between the measures in the pattern of variation across the cycle on a weekend compared with a weekday. This suggests that all the other measures of mood and performance are mirroring (to a lesser extent) the pattern of interaction observed in feelings of sociability. This is demonstrated in Figure 2-3 where all 11 of the mood and performance variables have been combined and mean score plotted in each phase of the cycle for weekend and weekday separately.

The consistency of this difference in weekend and weekday data indicates that something in the social environment of the weekend operates systematically to mediate the effect of the menstrual cycle. This finding is consistent with that of Rossi and Rossi (1977), who showed mood to be affected by both menstrual and social cycle. The present finding is a stronger illustration of the social mediation of the menstrual cycle, because the doubly repeated MANOVA analysis has made it possible simultaneously to make a comparison of the impacts of the social and menstrual cycles on women and to explore the interaction between the cycles.

In attempting to understand the interaction of the social week with the menstrual cycle the work of Schacter (1974) and Koeske and Koeske (1975) is useful. These researchers have shown that to experience an emotional state, one must have both a physical sensation and a cognitive construct (or explanation) for that sensation. The work of Schacter and Singer (1962) shows that the same sensation can be experienced as either a positive or a negative emotion depending on the cognitive construct that accompanies it. This provides insight into the

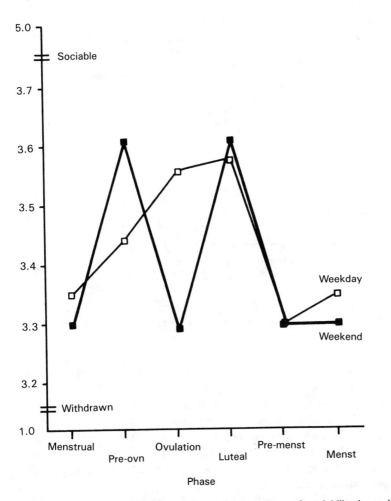

Figure 2-2 Weekend compared with weekday feelings of sociability in each phase of the cycle.

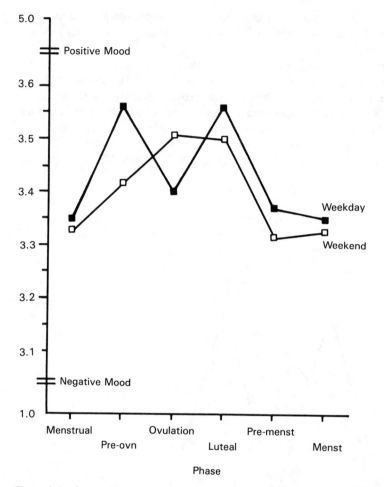

Figure 2-3 Comparison of weekday and weekend mean scores of combined mood and performance measures in each phase of the cycle.

individual psychological mechanisms that help to explain the diversity of human reactions to sensory experiences. The question of sociological interest is how competing explanations (cognitive constructs) emerge and become the framework through which bodily sensations are experienced and understood. In particular, researchers must look to the social context in addition to psychological explanations to understand how the menstrual cycle has become an interpretive framework through which the meanings and significance of women's bodily sensations are experienced.

I would contend that an excessive focus on the menstrual cycle as a determinant of women's behavior and capabilities has developed in the medical/

scientific literature and in popular culture during the 60 years since reproductive hormones were discovered. The overwhelmingly negative orientation of this focus had equated the menstrual cycle with illness and disability. The menstrual cycle has become synonymous in popular culture with PMS. The fact that this illness model of the menstrual cycle has been internalized by women became glaringly obvious in recruiting women to participate in this study. On each occasion I would describe the aim of my research as an attempt to understand different women's menstrual cycle experiences, only to be *heard* to say that I was studying PMS or "menstrual problems." The initial response of innumerable women was "I wouldn't be any use; I don't have period problems," or more tellingly *"I'm lucky,* I don't have any trouble at all. . . . I don't even know when it (my period) is coming." I was able to recruit many such women to the study by re-emphasizing that I was interested in the variety of ordinary women's experiences. However, the automatic equating of the menstrual cycle with "problems" of PMS demonstrated the extent to which women have internalized the cultural construct. They expect the cycle to have a negative impact and, if they don't experience problems, they describe themselves as the "lucky" exception to the rule. The results of my study, which show an interaction between the social cycle and the menstrual cycle, can be understood in the light of social expectations about negative menstrual cycle effects.

DISCUSSION

This study suggests that individual women continually filter their physical sensations through two competing interpretive frameworks—according to which phase of the cycle she believes herself to be in and according to whether it is a weekend or weekday. These cognitive constructs operate at a background, subliminal level rather than as conscious considerations. There is some evidence that when the salience of the menstrual cycle is increased so is the likelihood that sensations will be experienced and attributed to the cycle rather than to other factors. The two phases of the cycle that are emphasized in the social construction of cycle disorder are the menstrual and premenstrual phases. Therefore, bodily sensations would likely be attributed to the menstrual cycle in these phases as they are easily identified and have strong social expectations. It would follow that during the menstrual and premenstrual phases sensations are likely to be experienced more negatively regardless of the day of the week.

During phases of the cycle when there are less identifiable bodily sensations and when the menstrual cycle is not presumed to specifically affect behavior, the social context of weekday and weekend is likely to be more salient and, therefore, influential. For example, the preovulation phase is marked by the cessation of menstrual bleeding and is likely to be experienced positively, since it is free from the negative connotations (and/or sensations) of menstruation.

Figure 2-3 confirms that preovulation is experienced more positively, particularly when it coincides with the weekend.

Ovulation is a phase that is less easily anticipated or identified than other phases of the cycle, yet it is characterized by quite marked hormonal and biochemical fluctuations. Bodily sensations that accompany these fluctuations are less likely to be attributed to the menstrual cycle than to social factors. Although ovulation is a time of heightened physiological arousal, it remains a matter of conjecture as to why this physical state and the sensations that accompany it are interpreted more negatively when experienced in the social context of the weekend than when occurring on a weekday. It may be that the physiological arousal during ovulation facilitates the sort of interaction and emotion suited to the structured and "goal-oriented" weekday context. Thus ovulation is experienced positively on weekdays, whereas in the less structured weekend environment, when activities and interactions are more variable and negotiated, the heightened arousal of ovulation is experienced negatively.

A complex interaction is occurring between social and physiological factors at different phases of the menstrual cycle. This finding indicates the need for a more sophisticated understanding of the way in which bodily experiences are mediated by social factors. This study provides further challenge to a simplistic biodeterminist model of the menstrual cycle. It also indicates the need to reassess much of the accepted wisdom about the effects of the menstrual cycle. Such a reassessment should include a sociological investigation of the role that medico/scientific and lay concepts of the menstrual cycle play in the ongoing negotiation of gender.

REFERENCES

Australian Bureau of Statistics (1981). *Cross classified characteristics of persons and dwellings—South Australia: 1981 Census of Population and Housing*. Adelaide, South Australia: Australian Government Printer.

DSM-III-R. (1987): American Psychiatric Association, Working Group to Revise DSM-III. (1987). *Diagnostic and Statistical Manual of Mental Disorders, 3rd Edition Revised*. Washington, DC: Author.

Englander-Golden, P., Sonleitener, F. J., Whitmore, M., & Corbley, G. (1986). Social and menstrual cycles: Methodological and substantive findings. In V. Olesen & N. F. Woods (Eds.), *Culture, society, and menstruation*. Washington, DC: Hemisphere Publishing Corporation.

Englander-Golden, P., Whitmore, M. R., & Dienstbier, R. A. (1978). Menstrual cycle as a focus of self-reports of moods and behaviors. *Motivation and Emotion, 2*, 75–86.

Koeske, R. K., & Koeske, G. F. (1975). An attributional approach to moods and the menstrual cycle. *Journal of Personality and Social Psychology, 31*, 474–478.

Gannon, L. (1981). Evidence for a psychological etiology of menstrual disorders: A critical review. *Psychological Reports, 48*, 287–294.

Laws, S. (1983). The sexual politics of pre-menstrual tension. *Women's Studies International Forum, 6*(1), 19–31.

McIntosh, J. E. A., Matthews, C. D., Crocker, J. M., Broom, T. J., & Cox, L. W. (1980). Predicting the lutenizing hormone surge: Relationship between the duration of the follicular and luteal phases and the length of the human menstrual cycle. *Fertility and Sterility, 34*(2), 125–130.

Moos, R. H. (1968). The development of a menstrual distress questionnaire. *Psychosomatic Medicine, 30,* 853–867.

Moos, R. H. (1985). *Perimenstrual symptoms: A manual and overview of research with the menstrual distress questionnaire.* Stanford, CA: Stanford University Press.

Parlee, M. B. (1974). Stereotypic beliefs about menstruation. A methodological note on the Moos menstrual distress questionnaire and some new data. *Psychosomatic Medicine, 36*(3), 229–240.

Parlee, M. B. (1982). Change in mood and activation levels during the menstrual cycle in experimentally naive subjects. *Psychology of Women Quarterly, 7*(2), 119–131.

Rossi, A., & Rossi, E. (1977). Body time and social time: Mood patterns by menstrual cycle and day of the week. *Social Science Research, 6,* 273–308.

Ruble, D. N., & Brooks-Gunn, J. (1979). Menstrual symptoms: A social cognitive analysis. *Journal of Behavioral Medicine, 12*(2), 171–194.

Schacter, S. (1974). The interaction of cognitive and physiological determinants of emotional state. In P. Leiderman & D. Shapiro (Eds.), *Psychobiological approaches to social behavior.* Stanford, CA: Stanford University Press.

Schacter, S., & Singer, J. E. (1962). Cognitive social and physiological determinants of emotional state. *Psychological Review, 69,* 379–399.

Taylor, J. W. (1979). The timing of menstruation-related symptoms assessed by a daily symptom rating scale. *Acta Psychiatrica Scandinavica, 60,* 87–105.

Wilcoxon, L. A., Schrader, S. L., & Sherif, C. W. (1976). Daily reports of activities, life events, moods and somatic changes during the menstrual cycle. *Psychomatic Medicine, 38,* 399.

Wood, C., Larsen, L., & Williams, R. (1979). Menstrual characteristics of 2,343 women attending the Shepherd Foundation. *Australian and New Zealand Journal of Obstetrics and Gyneacology, 19,* 107.

Chapter 3

An Exploratory Study of the Menstrual Euphemisms, Beliefs, and Taboos of Head Start Mothers

Janice J. Jurgens and Bethel A. Powers

INTRODUCTION

The stimulus for this study originated in clinical practice. The questions that women asked, their statements about the menstrual process, and their use of menstrual euphemisms aroused a curiosity about the beliefs and taboos that might underlie and give meaning to what they were saying.

There is a dearth of research conducted within the United States about menstrual euphemisms, beliefs, and taboos. Much of the research is restricted to ethnic groups (Abel & Joffe, 1950; Devereux, 1950, Kay, 1981, Scott, 1975; Snow & Johnson, 1977). The literature suggests that menstrual beliefs and taboos may affect body image, self-esteem, perceptions of illness and wellness, diet, contraceptive choice, unplanned pregnancies, medical care, sexual activity, daily routines, self-care habits, and employment of women (Kay, 1981; Patterson & Hale, 1985; Roberts & Garling, 1981; Scott, 1975; Snow & Johnson, 1977).

The study reported here suggests that menstrual beliefs and taboos are not limited by ethnic, socioeconomic, and educational boundaries but rather cut across them. Head Start mothers were selected as subjects because they were accessible to the researcher and did not represent one particular ethnic group. Even though Head Start mothers are economically disadvantaged, they may not have been so in the past or intend to remain in this circumstance for long. The 13 women in this study had different educational and ethnic backgrounds; all but 1 woman were the third or fourth generation to be born in the United States. It may be speculated, then, that menstrual euphemisms, beliefs, and taboos that affect the well-being of women are more pervasive in our society than is presently recognized. Such an orientation might broaden research efforts in this area.

RESEARCH DESIGN AND METHOD

The 13 women participating in this study responded to a notice about the research that was placed in a Head Start newsletter, which was sent to 98 families. Initially 16 women volunteered.

Feminist methodology (MacPherson, 1983; Webb, 1984) was used in this descriptive study. This method involved a shared, nonhierarchical relationship between the interviewer and the interviewee in which the interviewer is prepared to invest personally in the interview by sharing information and answering the participant's questions. The interview schedule consisted of 16 structured questions eliciting biographical, gynecological, and obstetrical data and 15 open-ended questions about menstrual euphemisms, beliefs, and taboos.

The time allotment for each interview was 1 hr; however, flexibility was maintained so sufficient time was available for the interviewee to respond to all 15 open-ended questions and discuss her own experiences. Questions that were asked by the interviewees were addressed at the end of the interviews. If only a short response was needed, an answer was given at the time the question was asked. All the interviews were tape recorded and later transcribed. The responses to the open-ended questions were analyzed for unique or recurring themes.

This report summarizes findings from the open-ended conversations with the women; however, space will not allow for detailed examples of the richness of data obtained by this method.

FINDINGS

This section reports data concerning menstrual euphemisms, beliefs, and taboos.

Menstrual Euphemisms

The use of menstrual euphemisms may indicate reticence in dealing openly with the topics of menstruation and menopause (Ernster, 1975; McKeever, 1984; Weideger, 1976). When speaking with friends and family about menstruation, only one subject said that she sometimes used the word menstruation. The most commonly used menstrual euphemisms denote time and regularity (e.g., "period," "monthly," "that time"). Less frequently used euphemisms were those expressing ill health (e.g., "the curse," "the problem") or a visitor (e.g., "my friend"). The 13 women did not use but had heard euphemisms denoting the color red (e.g., "red flag days," "the reds,") and menstrual products (e.g., "on the rag"). As was found in previous research (Snowden & Christian, 1983), the women used the word menstruation or less vivid euphemisms that denote time and regularity when conversing with health care professionals. When discussing menopause, the euphemism "change of life" was frequently mentioned. Of the 13 women in this study, 4 said they had never talked about menopause, 2 had never heard menopause discussed, and 2 had heard the topic of menopause discussed once.

Menstrual Beliefs

Two menstrual beliefs concerning the purpose of menstruation were found among the women: (1) that menstruation is for pregnancy and (2) that it exists to cleanse the body of impurities. When asked what they believe causes menstruation to occur, 3 women did not know. Two women gave a somewhat technically accurate description of the menstrual cycle. Many believe that menstruation is caused by the release and bursting of ova. This belief may explain why all but 4 women believe that conception is most likely to occur close to the time of menstruation. Nine women believe that a change in their menstrual flow, lighter or heavier, is an indication of a health problem.

With the exception of 4 women who stated they had no knowledge about menopause, the beliefs expressed concerning the causes of menopause were that it is a result of hormonal changes, that the female body becomes too old to reproduce, and that it is God's wish.

That the moon affects behavior, menstrual cycles, or pregnancy are beliefs that 10 women had heard. Of these 10 women, 2 are absolutely certain of the moon's effects, and 4 think there may be some truth to what they heard.

When asked what their partners believe to be true about menstruation, 6 women said they had never discussed menstruation with them. Attitudes and not beliefs were expressed. Some said their partners think menstruation is disgusting and/or that it is a disruption of their sexual relationships.

Menstrual Taboos

The women mentioned numerous menstrual taboos. The salient theme found throughout the interviews was the need to avoid uncleanliness during menstruation. Most of the women always or sometimes douche after their menses so they feel clean.

All the women change their usual activities or practices to some extent during and following menstruation. Even though some of the women had been told not to bathe, shower, or wash their hair when menstruating, they do engage in these activities. Some think it is healthier to take baths, and others, showers.

Five women do not participate in strenuous activity or exercise during menstruation for fear that their health will be harmed. The 9 women who do not swim during their menses also avoided using tampons. Two women expressed the belief that cold water is harmful.

One woman avoids walking with bare feet on cold floors. Another did so until she tested the taboo and found that she suffered no ill effects. Only 1 woman avoids cold drinks and foods. Another said she had heard that hot drinks increase the flow, but does not believe it to be true.

Another woman does not garden, can, and bake because she believes the food would spoil. One woman does not cook because she believes the food does not taste good. Another woman cooks only if she has taken a shower or bath that day.

Until she was almost 30 years old, one woman said she did not shave her legs when menstruating. A friend told her that shaving was not harmful so she started shaving.

Four women only socialize within the family during their menses. Heavy menses, emotional discomfort, and feeling unclean were the reasons they gave.

For 10 women sexual intercourse during mensis is taboo because it is thought to be generally objectionable. Other reasons that they avoid intercourse during menses are that it is messy or harmful, affects the menses, there is risk of conception, the partner refuses, and religion prohibits it.

Most of the women prefer not to have a pelvic examination during menstruation. They think it is offensive for the examiner and themselves. Three of the 13 women stated that their doctors would not or preferred not to examine them if they were menstruating.

IMPLICATIONS

This nursing research has implications for all professionals who are involved in the health care of women, educational curricula, or research about women.

Clinical Practice

Making a conscious effort to avoid using euphemisms can help patients become accustomed to and more comfortable with menstrual events and products being called by name. Like their patients, some clinicians use euphemisms because of habit or custom, which probably originated out of feelings of embarrassment or shame. As one author (Weideger, 1976, pp. 3–4) wrote, "We are ashamed of menstruation and menopause. . . . This belief is reflected in our language—we don't call these events directly by name."

Understanding the legacy of menstrual beliefs and taboos and examining one's own beliefs prevents perpetuating misinformation. For example, women can be reassured that menstrual cycle variability is normal, that menstrual blood is not offensive or unclean, that pelvic examinations during menstruation are not taboo, and that activities or routines need not be restricted. Although some beliefs and taboos may be harmless, it is important to identify those that are potentially injurious and to offer alternatives that will not violate cultural and religious values that are important to patients. By providing information, clinicians can counteract the stigma, fear, and confusion that so many women feel about their bodies.

The health care system is partly responsible for women's misconceptions and discomforts about their bodies. Medical literature reflects and reinforces negative images and promulgates false information regarding natural female processes, which have often been addressed within the idiom of "disease" and "dysfunction." Instead of allowing specious theories, beliefs, and taboos to dominate the attitudes toward and the treatment of women's health care needs, clinicians must work forcefully to bring about needed changes.

Education

Medical and nursing students should be encouraged to understand their own and their patients' menstrual beliefs and taboos. Teaching only reproductive anatomy and physiology does not enlighten the student about the many variables that affect this physiological process and women's health needs.

The female physiological process is a continuum that begins before birth, really at the time of conception, and persists and changes throughout the lifetime of every woman. Instead of dividing females' lives into separate events of premenarche, menarche, menstruation, pregnancy, and menopause, educational programs must emphasize the interrelatedness of these events. Indeed, pregnancy is the only event that is openly discussed and prized by society. Nursing curricula that subsume women's health care issues under the heading of "maternal-child health" reflect this bias.

Research

Researchers who desire to be agents for social change and work for the betterment of humanity could consider becoming more involved in feminist research, which as MacPherson (1983, p. 19) stated "is grounded in women's actual experiences and is closely related to social change." One of the characteristics of current feminist research is choice of topics that not only affect women but also have been shrouded in silence (MacPherson, 1983). Certainly in the United States menstrual beliefs and taboos have been shrouded in silence. Researchers should become involved in studying menstruation—a process that has a pervasive influence on all women's lives.

REFERENCES

Abel, T., & Joffe, N. (1950). Cultural backgrounds of female puberty. *American Journal of Psychotherapy, 4,* 90–113.

Devereux, G. (1950). The psychology of feminine genital bleeding: An analysis of Mohave Indian puberty and menstrual rites. *International Journal of Psychoanalysis, 30*(4), 237–257.

Ernster, V. (1975). American menstrual expressions. *Sex Roles, 1*(1), 3–13.

Kay, M. (1981). Meanings of menstruation to Mexican American women. In P. Komnenich, P. McSweeney, J. Noack, & N. Elder (Eds.), *The menstrual cycle: Research and implications for women's health, Vol. 2* (pp. 114–123). New York: Springer.

MacPherson, K. (1983). Feminist methods: A new paradigm for nursing research. *Advances in Nursing Science, 5*(2), 17–24.

McKeever, P. (1984). The perpetuation of menstrual shame: Implications and directions. *Women and Health, 9*(4), 33–47.

Patterson, E., & Hale, E. (1985). Making sure: Integrating menstrual care practices into activities of daily living. *Advances in Nursing Science, 7*(3), 18–31.

Roberts, S., & Garling, J. (1981). The menstrual myth revisited. *Nursing Forum, 20*(30), 267–273.

Scott, C. (1975). The relationship between beliefs about the menstrual cycle and choice of fertility regulating methods within five ethnic groups. *International Journal of Gynecology and Obstetrics, 13,* 105–109.

Snow, L., & Johnson, S. (1977). Modern day menstrual folklore: Some clinical implications. *Journal of the American Medical Association, 237*(25), 2736–2739.

Snowden, R., & Christian, B. (Eds.). (1983). *Patterns and perceptions of menstruation: A World Health Organization international collaborative study in Egypt, India, Indonesia, Jamaica, Mexico, Pakistan, Philippines, Republic of Korea, United Kingdom, and Yugoslavia.* New York: St. Martin's Press.

Webb, C. (1984). Feminist methodology in nursing research. *Journal of Advanced Nursing, 9*(3), 249–256.

Weideger, P. (1976). *Menstruation and menopause: The physiology and psychology, the myth and the reality.* New York: A. A. Knopf.

Chapter 4

Menstrual Effects
on Neuroendocrine Measures

Daniel J. Cardona, Rajiv Tandon,
Roger F. Haskett, and John F. Greden

INTRODUCTION

Interest in the relationship between neuroendocrine fluctuations and psychological changes through the menstrual cycle is increasing. Although menstrual changes in the activity of gonadal steroids are well documented (Yen, 1980; Schnatz, 1985), menstrual changes in the activity of other endocrine systems are less well studied. Gonadal steroids modulate the activity of multiple central neurotransmitter systems (McEwen, Biegon, & Fischette, 1984); consequently, a researcher might expect menstrual changes in the activity of these neurotransmitters. Furthermore, emotional and behavioral changes are associated with specific phases of the menstrual cycle (Moos et al., 1969; Abramowitz, Baker, & Fleischer, 1982; Endicott, Halbreich, Schact & Nee, 1985; Backstrom, Sanders, & Leask, 1983); these psychological changes in turn have been related to neurotransmitter and neuroendocrine changes (Halbreich & Endicott, 1985). In this chapter, we will review the evidence for alterations in the activity of various neurotransmitter and endocrine systems throughout the menstrual cycle and present data indicating that hypothalamo-pituitary-adrenal (HPA) axis function, as reflected in the dexamethasone suppression test (DST) varies with phase of the menstrual cycle (Tandon, Cardona, Haskett, Alcser, & Greden, in press).

Menstrual Fluctuations in Central Neurotransmitters

The activity of various neurotransmitter systems appears to fluctuate throughout the menstrual cycle and is perhaps best viewed with reference to the ovulatory phase; most transmitters tend to have maximal or minimal activity in this phase. Estrogens contribute to menstrual changes in monoamine and other neurotransmitter systems by influencing neurotransmitter biosynthesis, turnover, and reuptake and by modulating receptor function.

For instance, with regard to the noradrenergic system, it appears that there is decreased norepinephrine (NE) synthesis and turnover and increased NE metabolism in the periovulatory period. Plasma activity of dopamine beta-hydroxylase (DBH), an enzyme that converts dopamine to norepinephrine, is found to be minimal in the periovulatory phase and maximal at the onset of menses (Redmond, Murphy, & Baulu, 1975). From a periovulatory trough, urinary levels of NE increase throughout the luteal phase until they peak at menstruation (Feichtinger et al., 1980). Platelet alpha-2 receptors show a similar pattern; maximal yohimbine binding occurs at menses (Jones et al., 1983). In contrast, platelet monoamine oxidase (MAO) activity is maximal at ovulation and minimal at menses (Redmond et al., 1975). These findings suggest that functional NE activity is lowest in the periovulatory phase (although there is an ovulatory peak related to the luteinizing hormone surge), increases throughout the luteal phase, and peaks during the menstrual phase.

Similarly, data suggest that the activity of other central neurotransmitters may vary as a function of menstrual phase. It appears that indices of dopaminergic (DA) activity are lowest during the periovulatory period and highest in the late-luteal phase (Ropert, Quigley, & Yen, 1984; Kletzky & Shangold, 1986). However, indices of serotonergic (5-HT) activity appear to be higher in the periovulatory phase in comparison to the perimenstrual phase (Tam, Mo-Yin, & Lee, 1985).

Neurotransmitters regulate the activity of endocrine systems, and these effects are summarized in Table 4-1.

Menstrual Fluctuations in Neuroendocrine Parameters

As with neurotransmitter systems, menstrual patterns of hormonal changes are best seen with reference to the periovulatory phase. Levels of gonadotrophic hormones and estrogens rise throughout the follicular phase, peak around ovulation, and then fall throughout the luteal phase to a nadir around menses. Progesterone levels tend to peak later, during the midluteal phase, and decline during the premenstrual period. Although menstrual cycle fluctuations in these hormones are well documented, menstrual changes in the activity of other neuroendocrine parameters are not. Such changes seem likely in view of the interactions of the hypothalamo-pituitary-gonadal axis with other hormonal systems

Table 4-1 Neurotransmitter Effects on Pituitary Hormone Secretion in Humans

	GH	Prolactin	TSH	ACTH	LH/FSH
Norepinephrine					
Alpha	↑	0	0	↑	0
Beta	↓	0	0	↓	0
Dopamine	↑	↓	↓	(↓)	↓(↑)
Serotonin	↑	↑	(↓)	↑	?
Acetylcholine	↓(↑)	?	?	↑	?
GABA	↑	↑	?	?	?
Enkephalin	↑	↑	(0)	(↓)	(↓)

↓, stimulates; ↓, inhibits; 0, no effect; ( ), suggestive effect; ?, unknown.

and in view of menstrual changes in the activity of various neurotransmitters, which in turn influence neuroendocrine activity (Table 4-1).

Growth hormone (GH) levels tend to rise throughout the follicular phase to peak levels at ovulation and then decline throughout the luteal phase to minimum levels at menses (Gennazini, Lemarchand-Beraud, Aubert, & Felber, 1975; Guidoux, Garnier, & Schimpff, 1986). The growth hormone response to insulin, apomorphine, clonidine, and other stimulatory agents tends to be enhanced in the periovulatory period in comparison with the menstrual period (Frantz & Rabkin, 1965; Merimee & Feinberg, 1971; Matussek, Ackenheil, & Herz, 1984; Hoehe, 1988). Similarly, the prolactin response to TRH and other stimulatory agents tends to be greater in the periovulatory period (Hoehe, 1988). Although serum TSH and T-3 levels are unchanged throughout the menstrual cycle (Weeke & Hansen, 1975), the TSH response to TRH (TRH stimulation test) tends to be blunted during the periovulatory and luteal phases. Plasma melatonin activity is minimal around ovulation and rises throughout the luteal phase (Arendt, 1978; Brun, Claustrat, & David, 1987), whereas beta-endorphin levels show the opposite pattern of a peak in the periovulatory phase and a nadir around menses (Wehrenberg, Wardlaw, Frantz, & Ferin, 1982; Hamilton & Gallant, 1989).

Hypothalamo-Pituitary-Adrenal (HPA) Axis Plasma ACTH levels reach a peak around the time of ovulation and a trough during menstruation (Gennazini, 1975; Gennazini et al., 1975; Burns, 1975). As mentioned, beta-endorphin levels follow a similar pattern, indicating that the activity of pro-opiomelanocortin (POMC, the precursor molecule of both ACTH and beta-endorphin; Roberts & Herbert, 1977) is highest in the periovulatory phase and lowest around menstruation. Plasma cortisol levels may show an identical pattern (Gennazini et al., 1975; Tam et al., 1985), with levels rising throughout the follicular phase and falling throughout the luteal phase. Collins, Eneroth, and Langdren (1985) observed higher baseline urinary cortisol levels in the ovulatory phase as compared to the follicular and luteal phases, although this pattern was reversed following stress. Plasma aldosterone and 11-deoxycorticosterone show a similar pattern, although their levels peak somewhat later in the luteal phase (Parker, Winkel, Rush, Porter, & MacDonald, 1981; Schwartz & Abraham, 1975).

METHODS

In an effort to evaluate menstrual effects on the dexamethasone suppression test (DST), we analyzed the results of a 1-mg DST (Carroll et al., 1980), completed each week throughout one complete menstrual cycle in 25 inpatients with major depression (Tandon et al., in press). Patients with any endocrinological or other major medical disorders, severe weight loss, malnutrition, or dehydration were excluded, and none received opiates, steroids, tegretol, or any other drugs that can interfere with interpretation of the DST. The DST was performed by administering 1 mg of dexamethasone at 11:30 p.m. on day 1 and obtaining blood samples for cortisol assay at 4:00 p.m. and 11:00 p.m. the next day. Throughout this cycle, 14 of these patients received no medication; the remaining 11 received a constant dose of antidepressant throughout this cycle.

RESULTS

We found that the maximum postdexamethasone serum cortisol concentrations were lowest at menses (mean = 3.84 μg/dL at week 0), rose to 4.94 μg/dL at week 1, reached a peak at midcycle (7.61 μg/dL at week 2), declined minimally to 6.89 μg/dL at week 3, and decreased to 5.45 μg/mL at week 4. Twenty-one of the 25 inpatients showed this pattern. Ten subjects were consistently *suppressive* and nine were consistently *nonsuppressive* throughout the entire menstrual cycle, but 6 patients were DST nonsuppressors only in weeks 2 or 3 of their cycles. There was no difference between medication-free patients and those on constant medication. The mean maximal postdexamethasone cortisol levels and depression ratings (Hamilton Rating Scale for Depression, HRSD; Hamilton, 1960) at various stages of the menstrual cycle are illustrated in Figure 4-1. These findings were not explained by changes in Hamilton depression ratings, weight, or other known sources of variance in HPA function.

DISCUSSION

The menstrual pattern of postdexamethasone cortisol levels was similar to that noted previously for ACTH, beta-endorphin, basal cortisol, aldosterone, and 11-deoxycorticosterone; highest levels occurred in the periovulatory and early luteal phases and lowest levels around menstruation.

Although much of the reported menstrual cycle variation in central neurotransmitters and hormones is preliminary and requires confirmation, the data

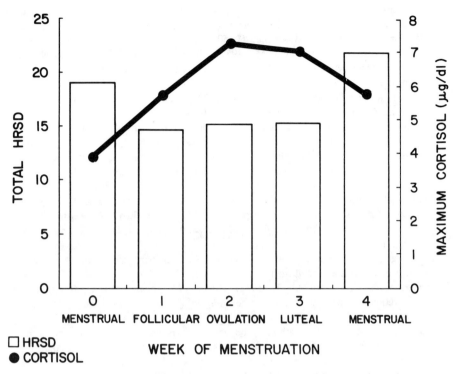

Figure 4-1 Mean maximal postdexamethasone cortisol and HRSD throughout the menstrual cycle.

suggest that many neuroendocrine systems fluctuate throughout the menstrual cycle. These oscillations in hormone secretion could be related to menstrual changes in the activity of various regulatory neurotransmitter systems. The precise relationship between these fluctuations and menstrual changes in mood and behavior deserve further attention in view of the observed influences of neurotransmitter and hormonal activity on mood and behavior. The menstrual cycle phase appears to be an important variable that warrants close consideration in the interpretation of results of various neuroendocrine tests in medicine.

REFERENCES

Abramowitz, E. S., Baker, A. H., & Fleischer, S. F. (1982). Onset of depressive psychiatric crises and the menstrual cycle. *American Journal of Psychiatry, 139,* 475–478.

Arendt, J. (1978). Melatonin assays in body fluids. *Journal of Neural Transmission* (suppl), *13,* 265–278.

Backstrom, T., Sanders, D. & Leask, R. (1983). Mood, sexuality, hormones, and the menstrual cycle. II. Hormone levels and their relationship to the premenstrual syndrome. *Psychosomatic Medicine, 45,* 503–507.

Brun, J., Claustrat, B., & David, M. (1987). Urinary melatonin, LH, oestradiol, and progesterone secretion during the menstrual cycle or in women taking oral contraceptives. *Acta Endocrinology* (Copenhagen), *116,* 145–149.

Burns, J. K. (1975). Variation in plasma ACTH levels during the human menstrual cycle. *Journal of Physiology* (London), *249,* 36P.

Carroll, B. J., Feinberg, M., Greden, J. F., et al. (1980). A specific laboratory test for the diagnosis of melancholia. *Archives of General Psychiatry, 28,* 15–22.

Collins, A., Eneroth, P., Landgren, B.-M. (1985). Psychoneuroendocrine stress responses and mood as related to the menstrual cycle. *Psychosomatic Medicine, 47,* 512–527.

Endicott, J., Halbreich, U., Schact, S., Nee, J. (1985). Affective disorder and premenstrual depression. In H. J. Osofsky & S. J. Blumenthal (Eds.), *Premenstrual syndrome: Current findings and future directions.* Washington, D.C.: American Psychiatric Press.

Feichtinger, W., Kemeter, P., Salzer, H., et al. (1980). Urinary catecholamine excretion in women with a normal menstrual cycle. *Wien Klin Wochenschrift, 92,* 365–368.

Frantz, A. G., & Rabkin, M. T. (1965). Effects of estrogen and sex differences on secretion of human growth hormone. *Journal of Clinical Endocrinology and Metabolism, 25,* 1470–1480.

Gennazini, A. R. (1975). Relationship between ACTH variations during the menstrual cycle and the adrenal androgen variations. *Hormone Research, 6,* 299–300.

Gennazini, A. R., Lemarchand-Beraud, T. H., Aubert, M. L., & Felber, J. P. (1975). Pattern of plasma ACTH, hGH and cortisol during the menstrual cycle. *Journal of Clinical Endocrinology and Metabolism, 41,* 431–437.

Guidoux, S., Garnier, P. E., & Schimpff, R. M. (1986). Effect of the variations of female sex hormones during the menstrual cycle upon serum somatomedin and growth-promoting activity. *Hormone Research, 23,* 31–37.

Halbreich, U., & Endicott, J. (1985). The biology of premenstrual changes: What do we really know? In H. J. Osofsky & S. J. Blumenthal (Eds.), *Premenstrual syndrome: Current findings and future directions.* Washington, D.C.: American Psychiatric Press.

Hamilton, M. (1960). Development of a scale for primary depressive illness. *British Journal of Social Clinical Psychology, 6,* 278–296.

Hamilton, J. A., & Gallant, S. (1988). Premenstrual symptom changes and plasma beta-endorphin/beta-lipotropin throughout the menstrual cycle. *Psychoneuroendocrinology, 13,* 505–514.

Hoehe, M. (1988). Influence of the menstrual cycle on neuroendocrine and behavioral responses to an opiate agonist in humans: Preliminary results. *Psychoneuroendocrinology, 13,* 339–344.

Kletzky, O. A., & Shangold, G. A. (1986). Variability and selectivity of anterior pituitary response to DA agonists throughout the normal menstrual cycle. *American Journal of Obstetrics and Gynecology, 154,* 362–367.

Jones, S. B., Bylund, D. B., Rieser, C. A. et al. (1983). Alpha-2 adrenergic receptor binding in human platelets. Alterations during the menstrual cycle. *Clinical Pharmacology Therapy, 34,* 90–96.

Matussek, N., Ackenheil, M., & Herz, M. (1984). The dependence of the clonidine growth hormone test on alcohol drinking habits and the menstrual cycle. *Psychoneuroendocrinology, 9,* 173–177.

McEwen, B. S., Biegon, A., & Fischette, C. T. (1984). Towards a neurochemical basis of steroid hormones action. In W. F. Ganong and L. Mortons (Eds.), *Frontiers in Neuroendocrinology.* New York: Raven Press.

Merimee, T. J., Fineberg, S. E. (1971). Studies of the sex based variation of human growth hormone secretion. *Journal of Clinical Endocrinology and Metabolism, 33,* 896–902.

Moos, R. H., Koppell, B. S., Melges, F. T., Yalom, I. D., Lunde, D. T., Clayton, R. B., Hamburg, D. A. (1969). Fluctuations in symptoms and moods during the menstrual cycle. *Journal of Psychosomatic Research, 13,* 37–44.

Parker, C. R., Winkel, C. A., Rush Jr., A. J., Porter, J. C. & MacDonald, P. C. (1981). Plasma concentrations of 11-deoxycorticosterone in women during the menstrual cycle. *Obstetrics and Gynecology, 58,* 26–30.

Redmond, D. E., Murphy, D. L., & Baulu, J. (1975). Menstrual cycle and ovarian hormone effects on plasma and platelet monoamine oxidase (MAO) and dopamine-beta-hydroxylase (DBH) activities in the rhesus monkey. *Psychosomatic Medicine, 37,* 417–428.

Roberts, J. L., & Herbert, E. (1977). Characterization of a common precursor to corticotropin and beta-lipotropin: Identification of beta-lipotropin peptides and their arrangement relative to corticotropin in the precursor synthesized in a cell-free system. *Proceedings of the National Academy of Science* (USA), *74,* 5300–5304.

Ropert, J. F., Quigley, M. E., & Yen, S. S. (1984). The dopaminergic inhibition of LH during the menstrual cycle. *Life Sciences, 34,* 2067–2073.

Schnatz, P. T. (1985). Neuroendocrinology and the ovulation cycle—advances and review. *Advanced Psychosomatic Medicine, 12,* 4–24.

Schwartz, U. D., & Abraham, G. E. (1975). Corticosterone and aldosterone levels during the menstrual cycle. *Obstetrics and Gynecology, 45,* 339–342.

Tam, W. Y. K., Mo-Yin, C., & Lee, P. H. K. (1985). Menstrual cycle and platelet 5-HT uptake. *Psychosomatic Medicine, 47,* 352–362.

Tandon, R., Cardona, D., Haskett, R. F., Alcser, K. & Greden, J. F. (in press). Menstrual cycle effects on dexamethasone suppression test in major depression. *Biological Psychiatry.*

Weeke, J., & Hansen, A. P. (1975). Serum TSH and serum T-3 levels during normal menstrual cycles and during cycles on oral contraceptives. *Acta Endocrinology* (Copenhagen), *79,* 431–438.

Wehrenberg, W. B., Wardlaw, S. L., Frantz, A. G., & Ferin, M. (1982). Beta-endorphin in hypophyseal blood: Variations throughout the menstrual cycle. *Endocrinology, 111,* 879–881.

Yen, S. S. (1980). Neuroendocrine regulation of the menstrual cycle. In D. T. Krieger & J. C. Hughes (Eds.), *Neuroendocrinology.* Sanderland, MA: Sinauer Association.

Chapter 5

Steroids and Brain Cell Activity During the Menstrual Cycle

John W. Phillis

INTRODUCTION

The relationship between steroid hormones and brain function has generally been considered to date from the point of view of feedback regulation of brain and anterior pituitary activity by the secretory products of endocrine glands. It is now accepted that steroid hormones exert this form of feedback control on pituitary secretion of their respective trophic hormones by binding to intracellular receptors and altering gene transcription in target cells within specific neuroendocrine structures (Pfaff & McEwan, 1983).

Steroids can also elicit very rapid changes in neuronal excitability, which are likely to be mediated by plasma-membrane bound receptors rather than by genomic mechanisms (Moss & Dudley, 1984). Although no interactions with specific components of the nerve cell membrane have as yet been firmly established, there are intriguing indications that glucocorticoids can affect the responses to putative neurotransmitters such as γ-aminobutyric acid (GABA), glutamic acid, acetylcholine, and the catecholamines (Janowsky & Davis, 1970; Simmonds, Turner, & Harrison, 1984; Majewska, Bisserbe, & Eskay, 1985). It is possible that steroid hormones exert their known hypnotic, anticonvulsant, and anesthetic actions in humans and animals by such interactions with the neurotransmitter systems of the central nervous system (Selye, 1942; Gyermek & Soyka, 1975; Hall, 1982; Pfaff & McEwan, 1983).

The influence of ovarian hormones on the excitability of neurons in the brain has long been the subject of considerable interest among neuropharmacologists. Since the pioneering studies of Woolley and Timiras (1962a, b), it has been known that estradiol can decrease electroshock seizure threshold in rats in a dose-dependent manner and that the threshold for the induction of electroshock convulsions in female rats is lowest during estrus. Furthermore, electroencephalographic seizures can be induced in cats by the topical application of estrogen on the cerebral cortex (Julian, Fowler, & Danielson, 1975). Conversely, 17β-estradiol has been described as having a hypnogenic action when injected intracerebroventricularly in rabbits (Paisley & Summerlee, 1984). Progesterone has been shown to increase electroshock seizure thresholds in animals (Spiegel & Wyeis, 1945) and decrease the frequency of spiking in an epileptic focus in the cat cerebral cortex (Landgren, Aasley, Backstrom, Dubrovsky, & Danielson, 1987).

Women characteristically attribute feelings of "well-being" and being "energetic" and "active" and the like to the late follicular phase of the menstrual cycle (Moos, Kopell, Melges, Yalom, Lunde, Clayton & Hamburg, 1969; Sanders, Warner, Backstrom, & Bancroft, 1983); this is a period of characteristic locomotor hyperactivity in rodents (Young & Fish, 1945; Quadagno, Shryne, Anderson, & Gorski, 1972). These indications of CNS activation contrast with the "fatigue" and depression associated with the luteal phase of the cycle (Moos et al., 1969; Sanders et al., 1983). It has been claimed that progestins in oral contraceptives are responsible for depression, lethargy, and reduced libido (Kane, Daly, Ewing, & Keller, 1967; Grant & Pryse-Davies, 1968). It is also alleged that falling progesterone levels are involved in the etiology of premenstrual tension (depression, tension, irritability, anxiety; Backstrom, 1977; Sanders et al., 1983) and for the instability of mood, anxiety, depression, and insomnia near term and following pregnancy (Kane et al., 1967; Treadway, Kane, Jarrahi-Zadeh, & Lipton, 1969).

Changes in epileptic seizure frequency occur during the menstrual cycle in some women: seizures are fewer during the luteal phase and increase as progesterone levels decline (catamenial epilepsy). These effects have been ascribed to the stabilizing action of progesterone on central excitability (Backstrom, 1977; Newmark & Penry, 1980; Mattson & Cramer, 1985). Thus, the presence of physiological concentrations of 17β-estradiol are associated with behavioral and neurophysiological manifestations of elevated brain excitability, whereas the elevated levels of progesterone during the luteal phase of the cycle can elicit a sedative type of activity.

Microiontophoretic and pressure ejection studies of the actions of estrogen on hypothalamic neuron activity have revealed excitatory and inhibitory effects of the steroid on medial preoptic-septal rat neurons, which occurred within seconds of the onset of application (Kelly, Moss, & Dudley, 1977; Poulain & Carette, 1981). 17β-estradiol has demonstrable excitant actions on pyramidal cells in a hippocampal slice preparation, increasing the amplitude of synaptically evoked field potentials (Foy & Teyler, 1983). Higher concentrations of 17β-estradiol had the opposite effect, depressing neuronal activity (Foy, Teyler, & Vardaris, 1982). Progesterone has been reported to depress single unit responses in the rat cerebral cortex (Komisaruk, McDonald, Whitmoyer, & Sawyer, 1967).

ADENOSINE

Interest in the potential involvement of adenosine in the depressant actions of steroids arose from preliminary observations that various steroids, including 17β-estradiol and progesterone, were potent inhibitors of the uptake of adenosine by rat brain cortical synaptosomes (Phillis & Wu, 1981). Further studies confirmed that 17β-estradiol and progesterone exhibited a competitive inhibition of adenosine uptake into cortical synaptosomes with K_1 values of 0.05 μM and 0.34 μM, respectively (Phillis, Bender, & Marszelec, 1985). Progesterone also inhibited adenosine uptake into cultured neurons and astrocytes with IC_{50} values of 10.2 μM and 5.0 μM, respectively (A.S. Bender, personal communication; cited in Phillis, 1986).

Adenosine, a naturally occurring compound in the brain, is a potent depressant of the firing of central neurons. It inhibits activity primarily by depressing the release of neurotransmitters from presynaptic nerve terminals and by a direct hyperpolarizing action on central neurons (Phillis & Wu, 1981; Stone, 1981; Dunwiddie, 1985). Adenosine appears to be released from neurons into the interstitial space both in the form of a precursor, adenosine 5-triphosphate (ATP), which is rapidly metabolized into adenosine, and directly as adenosine itself. Release of ATP is likely to be vesicular and calcium-dependent, whereas release of adenosine is mediated by a membrane transporter. There is ample evidence to suggest that the excitability of central neurons is normally modulated by extracellular adenosine. The stimulant methylxanthines, caffeine and theophylline, antagonize the depressant effects of adenosine, and this action explains their CNS stimulant properties. Conversely, agents that prevent the removal of adenosine from the extracellular space, by inhibiting its uptake or deamination, have potent depressant actions on neuronal firing (Phillis & Wu, 1981). Adenosine can therefore be considered as a modulator of neuronal excitability, and agents that potentiate or antagonize the actions of adenosine would be expected to affect brain excitability.

PROGESTOGENS

Progesterone concentrations in the plasma of female rats range between 2 ± 1 ng/ml and 46.7 ng/ml (10^{-8} M to 1.5×10^{-7} M) at various stages of the estrous cycle (Butcher, Collins, & Fugo, 1974). Plasma concentrations in women can reach 18 ng/ml (5.7×10^{-8} M) during the luteal phase of the menstrual cycle and in excess of 600 ng/ml during pregnancy (Backstrom, 1977). Progesterone accumulates in several regions of the central nervous system, including the cerebral cortex (Wade, Harding, & Feder, 1973; Backstrom, 1977) where concentrations can be four times those in plasma. The concentrations of progesterone in the brain therefore would be sufficient, during the luteal phase, to cause a 25 to 40% inhibition of adenosine uptake into cerebral cortical nerve endings and should significantly enhance adenosine levels in the extracellular space.

The abilities of progesterone and several synthetic progestins to potentiate the depressant effects of adenosine were tested in experiments on rat cerebral cortical neurons. When applied iontophoretically from one barrel of a multiple-barrelled micropipette, progesterone potentiated (by inhibitory actions of adenosine ejected from another barrel of the micropipette) the spontaneous firing of rat cerebral neurons (Phillis et al., 1985). Intravenously administered progesterone (200 μg/kg) depressed the spontaneous firing of cerebral cortical neurons and prolonged the mean duration of adenosine-evoked inhibitions by 56% (Phillis, 1986). Tests with 3 synthetic progestins (norethindrone, cyproterone, and pregnenolone sulfate) (Corpechot et al., 1983) revealed comparable enhancing actions on adenosine's depressant effects (Figure 5-1). Norethindrone, cyproterone, and pregnenolone sulfate failed to potentiate the depressant actions of an adenosine analog, adenosine 5'-N-ethylcarboxamide (NECA), which is not transported by the uptake system, confirming that the enhancement of adenosine's action was a result of inhibition of its removal from the extracellular space. Cyproterone and norethindrone had depressant effects on neuronal firing. Confirmation that this action involved adenosine was obtained by demonstrating antagonism with caffeine (Figure 5-2) (Phillis, 1986).

ESTROGENS

Plasma 17β-estradiol levels in human and rat plasma fluctuate during the estrous cycle, reaching peak concentrations of approximately 10^{-9} M before ovulation (Backstrom et al., 1976; Butcher et al., 1974).

When 17β-estradiol was applied on a number of spontaneously active rat cerebral cortical neurons, the most frequently observed responses were either a decrease in the rate of spontaneous firing (44%) occurring within 1–2 min of the onset of steroid application or the absence of any change in the spontaneous activity (47%) (Phillis & O'Regan, 1988). An increase in firing rate was observed with a few neurons (9%). Firing rates returned to control levels within a

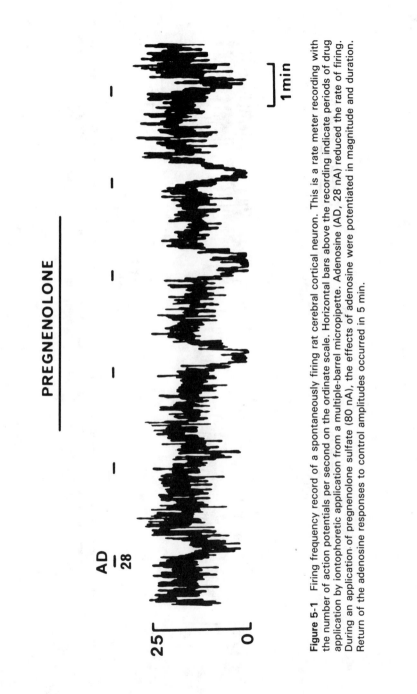

Figure 5-1 Firing frequency record of a spontaneously firing rat cerebral cortical neuron. This is a rate meter recording with the number of action potentials per second on the ordinate scale. Horizontal bars above the recording indicate periods of drug application by iontophoretic application from a multiple-barrel micropipette. Adenosine (AD, 28 nA) reduced the rate of firing. During an application of pregnenolone sulfate (80 nA), the effects of adenosine were potentiated in magnitude and duration. Return of the adenosine responses to control amplitudes occurred in 5 min.

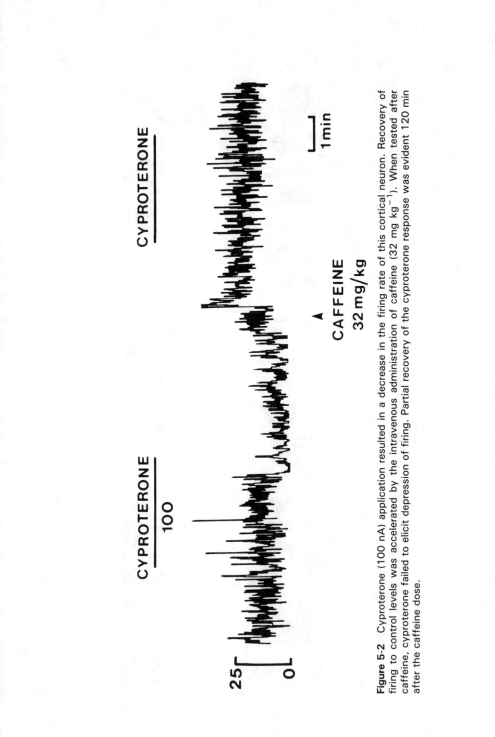

Figure 5-2 Cyproterone (100 nA) application resulted in a decrease in the firing rate of this cortical neuron. Recovery of firing to control levels was accelerated by the intravenous administration of caffeine (32 mg kg⁻¹). When tested after caffeine, cyproterone failed to elicit depression of firing. Partial recovery of the cyproterone response was evident 120 min after the caffeine dose.

few minutes of the cessation of steroid application. 17α-estradiol, a weak or inactive estrogen with no effect on reproductive function, was used as a control for the effects of the 17β-isomer. It also had a mild depressant action on the firing cerebral cortical neurons, which may have been a result of its weak ability to inhibit adenosine transport (Phillis et al., 1985).

For tests of their effects on purine-evoked depressions, the two steroids (17β- and 17α-estradiol) were applied in amounts that did not alter spontaneous firing. 17β-estradiol had both potentiative and antagonistic effects on adenosine-evoked inhibitions of spontaneous firing. To ascertain whether the potentiative effects of 17β-estradiol were a result of inhibition of adenosine transport, it was tested against NECA-evoked depression of firing. No potentiation of NECA was observed, but on 76% of the neurons tested 17β-estradiol antagonized NECA-evoked depressions (Phillis & O'Regan, 1988).

17α-estradiol potentiated adenosine's action on 50% of the neurons tested, but failed to antagonize adenosine- or NECA-evoked inhibition on any of the neurons tested. The ability to antagonize purine actions is apparently limited to the naturally occurring estrogen, 17β-estradiol. It appears that although both the 17α- and 17β-estradiols are able to inhibit adenosine transport, only the 17β-estrogen can act as an antagonist at the adenosine receptor.

Although 17β-estradiol concentrations in the extracellular fluid of the brain are unlikely to reach levels at which the activity of the adenosine transporter is compromised, they may be sufficient to antagonize the actions of endogenously released adenosine, exerting a caffeinelike stimulating action on the central nervous system. Such an action could account for the emotions attributed to the follicular phase of the menstrual cycle.

PREMENSTRUAL TENSION AND POSTPARTUM DEPRESSION

Premenstrual tension and postpartum depression share characteristic symptoms such as irritability, increased tension, and exhaustion; their occurrence coincides with a fall in circulating progesterone levels. The high progesterone levels in the early luteal phase and in pregnancy may lead to the development of a "dependency" on this natural anxiolytic. A sudden physiological drop in progesterone levels could evoke a "withdrawal syndrome" with associated symptoms such as anxiety and depression. This "withdrawal" effect would result from a combination of a reduction in the amount of extracellular adenosine, resulting from recovery of the transport of adenosine into nerve cells and glia, with a down-regulation of adenosine receptors in response to the elevated levels of extracellular adenosine at an earlier stage of the luteal phase.

There have been recent reports of a relationship between the consumption of the adenosine antagonist, caffeine, and the severity of premenstrual syndrome (PMS) in young women (Rossignol, 1985, 1989). Caffeine may exacerbate PMS by further reducing the diminished adenosinergic inhibitory tone in the central nervous system described earlier. Appropriate changes in caffeine consumption levels may help women to control the emotional fluctuations associated with the menstrual cycle. Caffeine intake should be sharply reduced during the 14- to 15-day period between day 1 of menstruation and ovulation, when progesterone levels are low and the rising 17β-estradiol levels enhance CNS excitability by blocking adenosine (in a caffeinelike manner). Caffeine intake would gradually be increased from day 15 to day 23 of the cycle, to counteract the adenosine-enhancing actions of progesterone, and then rapidly decreased again between days 23 and the onset of menstruation, when progesterone levels are falling. Careful management of the intake of caffeine along these lines may provide an appropriate strategy for controlling the emotional aspects of premenstrual syndrome.

CONCLUSIONS

Steroid actions on the CNS can be divided into slow genomic actions and rapid effects that are mediated through the plasma membrane. Modifications of adenosinergic inhibitory tone, resulting in enhanced (17β-estradiol) or reduced (progesterone) neuronal excitability, may represent important elements of the communication between the body and the brain, which is essential for appropriate integrated behavioral responses. In some instances, such as premenstrual syndrome or catamenial epilepsy, individual susceptibility to the changing levels of reproductive hormones may lead to imbalances between central excitation and inhibition with resultant psychological or neurological consequences. Manipulation of caffeine intake may provide a convenient and accessible route for the control of such imbalances.

REFERENCES

Backstrom, T. (1977). Estrogen and progesterone in relation to different activities in the central nervous system. *Acta Obstetrica et Gynecologica Scandinavica, 56*(Suppl. 66), 1–17.

Backstrom, T., Baird, D. T., Bancroft, J., Bixo, M., Hammarback, S., Sanders, D., Smith, S., & Zetterlund, B. (1983). Endocrinological aspects of cyclical mood changes during the menstrual cycle or the premenstrual syndrome. *Journal of Psychosomatic Obstetrics and Gynaecology, 2-1*, 8–20.

Backstrom, T., Bixo, M., Dubrovsky, B., Landgren, S., Lofgren, M., Norberg, L., Sorensen, M., & Wahlstrom, G. (1986). Brain excitability, steroid hormone and the menstrual cycle. In L. Dennerstein & I. Fraser (Eds.), *Hormones and Behavior* (pp. 137–142). Amsterdam: Elsevier Science Publishers.

Butcher, R. L., Collins, W., & Fugo, N. W. (1974). Plasma concentration of LH, FSH, prolactin, progesterone and estradiol 17-β throughout the 4-day estrous cycle of the rat. *Endocrinology, 94*, 1704–1708.

Corpechot, C., Synguelakis, M., Talha, S., Axelson, M., Sjovall, J., Vihko, R., Baulieu, E. E., & Robel, P. (1983). Pregnenolone and its sulphate ester in the rat brain. *Brain Research, 270*, 119–125.

Dunwiddie, T. V. (1985). The physiological role of adenosine in the central nervous system. *International Review of Neurobiology, 27*, 63–139.

Foy, M. R., & Teyler, T. J. (1983). 17-α-Estradiol and 17-β-estradiol in hippocampus. *Brain Research Bulletin, 10,* 735–739.

Foy, M. R., Teyler, T. J., & Vardaris, R. M. (1982). Δ^9-THC and 17β-estradiol in hippocampus. *Brain Research Bulletin, 8,* 341–345.

Grant, E., & Pryse-Davis, J. (1968). Effect of oral contraceptives on depressive mood changes and on endometrial monoamine oxidase and phosphatases. *British Medical Journal, 3,* 777–780.

Gyermek, L., & Soyka, L. F. (1975). Steroid anesthetics. *Anesthesiology, 42,* 331–344.

Hall, E. D. (1982). Glucocorticoid effects on central nervous excitability and synaptic transmission. *International review of Neurobiology, 23,* 165–195.

Janowsky, D. S., & Davis, J. M. (1970). Progesterone-estrogen effects on uptake and release of norepinephrine by synaptosomes. *Life Sciences, 9,* 525–531.

Julian, R. M., Fowler, G. W., & Danielson, M. G. (1975). The effects of antiepileptic drugs on estrogen-induced electrographic spike-wave discharge. *Journal of Pharmacology and Experimental Therapeutics, 193,* 647–656.

Kane, F. J., Daly, R. J., Ewing, J. A, & Keller, M. H. (1967). Mood and behavioral changes with progestational agents. *British Journal of Psychiatry, 113,* 265–268.

Kelly, M. J., Moss, R. L., & Dudley, C. A. (1977). The effects of microelectrophoretically applied estrogen, cortisol, and acetylcholine on medial preoptic septal unit activity throughout the estrous cycle of the female rat. *Experimental Brain Research, 30,* 53–64.

Komisaruk, B. R., McDonald, P. G., Whitmoyer, D. I., & Sawyer, C. H. (1967). Effects of progesterone and sensory stimulation on EEG and neuronal activity in the rat. *Experimental Neurology, 19,* 494–507.

Landgren, S., Aasley, J., Backstrom, T., Dubrovsky, B., & Danielson, E. (1987). The effect of progesterone and its metabolites on the interictal epileptiform discharge in the cat's cerebral cortex. *Acta Physiologica Scandinavica, 131,* 33–42.

Majewska, M. D., Bisserbe, J.-C., & Eskay, R. L. (1985). Glucocorticoids are modulators of GABA$_A$ receptors in brain. *Brain Research, 339,* 178–182.

Mattson, R. H., & Cramer, J. A. (1985). Epilepsy, sex hormones, and antiepileptic drugs, *Epilepsia, 26*(1), S40–S51.

Moos, R. H., Kopell, B. S., Melges, F. T., Yalom, I. D., Lunde, D. T., Clayton, R. B., & Hamburg, D. A. (1969). Fluctuations in symptoms and moods during the menstrual cycle. *Journal of Psychosomatic Research, 13,* 37–44.

Moss, R. L., & Dudley, C. A. (1984). Molecular aspects of the interaction between estrogen and the membrane excitability of hypothalamic cells. *Progress in Brain Research, 61,* 3–21.

Newmark, M. E., & Penry, J. K. (1980). Catamenial epilepsy. A review. *Epilepsia, 21,* 281–300.

Paisley, A. C., & Summerlee, A. J. S. (1981). Relationships between behavioral states and activity of the cerebral cortex. *Progress in Neurobiology, 22,* 155–184.

Pfaff, D. W., & McEwen, B. S. (1983). Actions of estrogens and progestins on nerve cells. *Science, 219,* 808–813.

Phillis, J. W. (1986). Potentiation of the depression by adenosine of rat cerebral cortical neurons by progestational agents. *British Journal of Pharmacology, 89,* 693–702.

Phillis, J. W., Bender, A. S., & Marszalec, W. (1985). Estradiol and progesterone potentiate adenosine's depressant action on rat cerebral cortical neurons. *General Pharmacology, 16,* 609–612.

Phillis, J. W., & O'Regan, M. H. (1988). Effects of estradiol on cerebral cortical neurons and their responses to adenosine. *Brain Research Bulletin, 20,* 151–155.

Phillis, J. W., & Wu, P. H. (1981). The role of adenosine and its nucleotides in central synaptic transmission. *Progress in Neurobiology, 16,* 187–239.

Poulain, P., & Carette, B. (1981). Pressure ejection of drugs on single neurons in vivo: Technical considerations and application to the study of estradiol effects. *Brain Research Bulletin, 7,* 33–40.

Quadagno, D. M., Shryne, J., Anderson, C., & Gorski, R. A. (1972). Influence of gonadal hormones in social, sexual, emergence and open field behavior in the rat, *Rattus norvegicus. Animal Behavior, 20,* 732–740.

Rossignol, A. M. (1985). Caffeine-containing beverages and premenstrual syndrome in young women. *American Journal of Public Health, 75,* 1335–1337.

Rossignol, A. M., Zhang, J., Chen, Y., Xiang, Z. (1989). Tea and premenstrual syndrome in the People's Republic of China. *American Journal of Public Health, 79,* 67–69.

Sanders, D., Warner, P., Backstrom, T., & Bancroft, J. (1983). Mood, sexuality, hormones and the menstrual cycle. 1. Changes in mood and physical state: Description of subjects and method. *Psychosomatic Medicine, 45,* 487–501.

Selye, H. (1942). Studies concerning the correlation between anesthetic potency, hormonal activity and chemical structure among steroid compounds. *Anesthesia and Analgesia, 21,* 41–47.

Simmonds, M. A., Turner, J. P., & Harrison, N. L. (1984). Interactions of steroids with GABA$_A$ receptor complex. *Neuropharmacology, 23,* 877–878.

Spiegel, E., & Wyeis, H. (1945). Anticonvulsant effects of steroids. *Journal of Laboratory and Clinical Medicine, 30,* 947–953.

Stone, T. W. (1981). Physiological roles for adenosine and ATP in the nervous system. *Neuroscience, 6,* 523–555.

Treadway, R. C., Kane, F. J., Jarrahi-Zadeh, A., & Lipton, M. A. (1969). A psychoendocrine study of pregnancy and puerperium. *American Journal of Psychiatry, 125,* 1380–1386.

Wade, G. N., Harding, C. F., & Feder, H. H. (1973). Neural uptake of [1, 2-^{3}H] progesterone in ovariectomized rats, guinea pigs and hamsters: Correlation with species differences in behavioral responsiveness. *Brain Research, 61,* 357–367.

Woolley, D. E., & Timiras, P. S. (1962a). The gonad-brain relationship: Effects of female sex hormones on electroshock convulsions in the rat. *Endocrinology, 70,* 196–209.

Woolley, D. E., & Timiras, P. S. (1962b). Estrous and circadian periodicity and electroshock convulsions in rats. *American Journal of Physiology, 202,* 379–382.

Young, W. C., & Fish, W. R. (1945). The ovarian hormones and spontaneous running activity in the female rat. *Endocrinology, 36,* 181–189.

Chapter 6

A First Attempt at Estimating Luteinizing Hormone Surge Onset Day at Midcycle

Cynthia Hedricks, Linda J. Piccinino, and J. Richard Udry

INTRODUCTION

A peak in coital behavior around ovulation in the female is a consistent finding across most mammalian species. The peak in coital behavior is often determined, to a large degree, by changes in female reproductive hormones. There is a lack of agreement among studies of humans, however, in whether the coital rate peaks around the expected time of ovulation (Udry & Morris, 1968, 1970; Spitz, Gold, & Adams, 1975; Bancroft, Sanders, Davidson, & Warner, 1983) and thus whether changes in women's hormones at midcycle affect human coital behavior.

Some of the discrepancy between these aforementioned studies may have resulted from the use of nonhormonal methods to estimate the time of ovulation, a methodological decision that can have a profound influence on the distribution of sexual behavior across the menstrual cycle (Morris & Udry, 1982). These investigators concluded that hormonal measures must be collected by

We greatly acknowledge the assistance of Thomas H. K. Chimbira, MD, Karin Gleiter, PhD, Jilane B. Matinga, SRN, SCM, Marilyn Maxwell, SRN, Mike Mbizvo, MPhil, Nancy Dole Runkle, MSPH, and Jian-yu Wang, MD.

those studying relationships between phase of the menstrual cycle and human sexual behavior.

Following this recommendation, we recently measured urinary luteinizing hormone (LH) and the incidence of menses and coitus in married women. Coital behavior was organized around LH surge onset, since this event is considered to be a better reference point for steroid hormone changes at midcycle than LH peak (Hoff, Quigley, & Yen, 1983; Yen, 1986). Coital rate of the sample increased almost steadily during the follicular phase of the menstrual cycle and peaked on LH surge onset day at midcycle (Hedricks, Piccinino, Udry, & Chimbira, 1987).

LH surge onset appears to be a biologically meaningful reference point from which to organize human coital behavior across the female's menstrual cycle. However, not all of our colleagues collect hormonal measures for determination of LH surge onset. The goal of this paper was an attempt to estimate LH surge onset day with a nonhormonal measure, menstrual cycle length. Cycle length was chosen because of the positive association between cycle length and follicular phase length (Sherman & Korenman, 1974; McIntosh, Matthews, Crocker, Broom, & Cox, 1980; Lenton, Landgren, Sexton, & Harper, 1984) and because it is simple, inexpensive, and noninvasive to collect. The validity of the nonhormonal estimate was tested on a sample for which urinary LH, cycle length, and coital behavior were available.

METHODS

Data from 24 healthy, noncontracepting married couples from Harare, Zimbabwe, were used. Daily morning urine specimens and daily reports of intercourse (yes/no) and menstruation (yes/no) were collected from the women for at least 90 days. Detailed information on recruitment, sample characteristics, and data collection and analysis have been reported previously (Hedricks et al., 1987).

Data from only one menstrual cycle per woman were used. The first day of menses was considered to be forward cycle day 1. Urinary LH values (Amerlex LH RIA kit, Amersham Corporation, Arlington Heights, IL) from forward cycle days 5 to 20 were used to determine the forward cycle day of LH surge onset and the forward cycle day of the LH peak. The day on which the LH value was the greatest was considered to be LH peak day. Counting backward 5 days from LH peak day, the day on which the LH level was $\geq 180\%$ of the level of the day before, was considered to be LH surge onset day. LH values in urine were matched with the coital report from the previous day, because LH activity in urine typically lags behind LH activity in plasma by about 1 day (Roger, Grenier, Houlbert, Castanier, Feinstein, & Scholler, 1980).

RESULTS

The mean length (and SD) of the 24 menstrual cycles was 26.71 (SD = 2.49) days. LH surge onset day ranged between forward cycle days 10 and 19, and on average occurred on forward cycle day 13.08 (SD = 2.15). There was a very strong positive correlation between LH surge onset day and cycle length (r = .75; $p < .0001$; Figure 6-1), whereas the correlation between *reverse* cycle day of LH surge onset and cycle length was less strong (r = .53; $p < .01$). The regression equation of LH surge onset day based on cycle length was: LH surge onset day ($\hat{Y}$) = $-4.21 + (0.65 \times$ cycle length).

For each of the 24 menstrual cycles, LH surge onset day was estimated using the above regression formula. In only six (25%) of the cycles was the estimated LH surge onset day the same day as the actual (observed) LH surge onset day. The distribution of coitus according to the estimated LH surge onset day is presented in Figure 6-2. Note that this method of estimation does not produce the significant peak in coital behavior that was found on the actual day of LH surge onset, or day 0 (Hedricks et al., 1987).

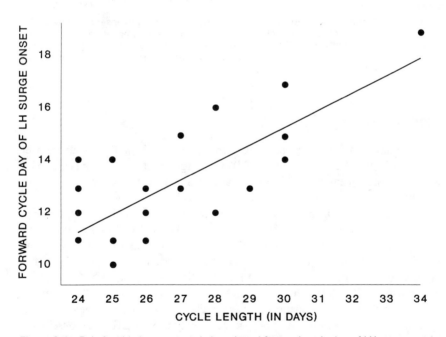

Figure 6-1 Relationship between cycle length and forward cycle day of LH surge onset. There was a highly significant, positive correlation between cycle length and forward cycle day of LH surge onset (r = .75; $p < .0001$).

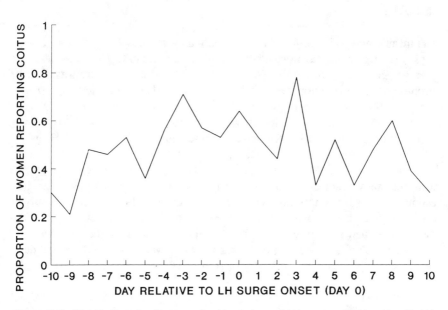

Figure 6-2 Distribution of coitus organized by estimated LH surge onset day (day 0). LH surge onset day (Ŷ) was estimated using the regression equation, $\hat{Y} = -4.21 + (0.65 \times \text{cycle length})$. The observed midcycle peak in coitus on LH surge onset day (Hedricks et al., 1987) was not apparent when LH surge onset day was estimated with this regression equation.

DISCUSSION

Coital behavior in human couples has been found to peak on the LH surge onset day at midcycle (Hedricks et al., 1987). LH surge onset day thus appears to be a biologically meaningful reference point from which to explore changes in human behavior across the female menstrual cycle.

Because not all investigators have available to them biological specimens from which to determine LH surge onset day, the goal of this report was to attempt to estimate LH surge onset day using a nonhormonal measure. Menstrual cycle length was used to estimate LH surge onset day, because of the close association between cycle length and follicular phase length (Sherman & Korenman, 1974; McIntosh et al., 1980; Lenton et al., 1984). Although there was a strong positive correlation between cycle length and LH surge onset day, cycle length alone was not sufficient to accurately predict LH surge onset day. The regression equation obtained resulted in an accurate prediction of LH surge onset day in only six (25%) of the cycles. Furthermore, the estimation did not yield the observed midcycle peak in coitus on LH surge onset day (Hedricks et al., 1987).

At present, we can offer no accurate estimation of LH surge onset day based on a nonhormonal measure. It is possible that improved accuracy in estimation might result from data on a larger sample size or from nonhormonal measures that were not included in the regression equation. Until a greater degree of accuracy is obtained using a nonhormonal method, we recommend a hormonal determination of LH surge onset when investigating whether human coital behavior increases around the time of ovulation in the female.

REFERENCES

Bancroft, J., Sanders, D., Davidson, D., & Warner, P. (1983). Mood, sexuality, hormones, and the menstrual cycle. III. Sexuality and the role of androgens. *Psychosomatic Medicine, 45,* 509–516.

Hedricks, C., Piccinino, L. J., Udry, J. R., & Chimbira, T. H. K. (1987). Peak coital rate coincides with onset of luteinizing hormone surge. *Fertility and Sterility, 48,* 234–238.

Hoff, J. D., Quigley, M. E., & Yen, S. S. C. (1983). Hormonal dynamics at midcycle: A re-evaluation. *Journal of Clinical Endocrinology and Metabolism, 57,* 792–796.

Lenton, E. A., Landgren, B.-M., Sexton, L., & Harper, R. (1984). Normal variation in the length of the follicular phase of the menstrual cycle: Effect of chronological age. *British Journal of Obstetrics and Gynaecology, 91,* 681–684.

McIntosh, J. E. A., Matthews, C. D., Crocker, J. M., Broom, T. J., & Cox, L. W. (1980). Predicting the luteinizing hormone surge: Relationship between the duration of the follicular and luteal phases and the length of the human menstrual cycle. *Fertility and Sterility, 34,* 125–130.

Morris, N. M., & Udry, J. R. (1982). Epidemiological patterns of sexual behavior in the menstrual cycle. In R. C. Friedman (Ed.), *Behavior and the Menstrual Cycle* (pp. 129–153). New York: Marcel Dekker, Inc.

Roger, M., Grenier, J., Houlbert, C., Castanier, M., Feinstein, M.-C., & Scholler, R. (1980). Rapid radioimmunoassays of plasma LH and estradiol-17β for the prediction of ovulation. *Journal of Steroid Biochemistry, 12,* 403–410.

Sherman, B. M., & Korenman, S. G. (1974). Hormonal characteristics of the human menstrual cycle throughout reproductive life. *Journal of Clinical Investigation, 55,* 699–706.

Spitz, C. J., Gold, A. R., & Adams, D. B. (1975). Cognitive and hormonal factors affecting coital frequency. *Archives of Sexual Behavior, 4,* 249–263.

Udry, J. R., & Morris, N. M. (1968). Distribution of coitus in the menstrual cycle. *Nature, 220,* 593–596.

Udry, J. R., & Morris, N. M. (1970). Effect of contraceptive pills on the distribution of sexual activity in the menstrual cycle. *Nature, 227,* 502–503.

Yen, S. S. C. (1986). The human menstrual cycle. In S. S. C. Yen & R. B. Jaffe (Eds.), *Reproductive Endocrinology* (pp. 200–236). Philadelphia: W. B. Saunders Company.

Chapter 7

Feminine Hygiene Considerations for the Space Environment

Barbara Shelden Czerwinski

INTRODUCTION

Envisioned for the 21st century is the United States space program's establishment of a permanent human presence in space on a space station and a moon colony. Midcentury humans will take part in an exploratory trip to Mars from the moon (Collins, 1988; Ride, 1987).

Vital to the achievement of the United States space goals will be human health management in the space environment. Later, there will be domestic application of aerospace technologies to improve the quality of life on Earth. Baseline human requirements will be developed to provide knowledge essential to the achievement of the space program's goals of extended human space

The author teaches undergraduate and graduate students and is completing doctoral-level research at Texas Woman's University—Houston. She has added to the personal hygiene database from a health maintenance perspective as a continuation of her work on the Space Station Personal Hygiene Study (SSPHS) (NASA contract NASA 9-17500-SSPHS 7708, August 1985 to July 1986). Based on work as a research analyst and a human test subject for two prime NASA contractors, opinions herein expressed are those of the author and do not reflect official positions of NASA or any other agency, corporation, or association.

inhabitation. Ground-based research is needed for space health management for preventive care (nonmedical measures) to preserve crew health (NASA, 1987).

As defined in this chapter, the aerospace environment pertains to flight within and outside the Earth's atmosphere. Hardware is equipment or fixtures that can be used repeatedly. Consumable products (space crew supplies) are usually used once and disposed of. By-products are additional products produced as waste from the products used on the body or human output or waste products (NASA, 1988).

OVERVIEW OF RESEARCH ON FEMININE HYGIENE IN SPACE

Human space travel requirements are based on standards from the Earth's environment and previous human space experiences. Space requirements are formulated from societal norms and engineering feasibility studies and from simulations that become standards. For example, humans require air, water, food, protection from radiation, and gravity to maintain life. United States space travel has been centered primarily on habitability considerations for 84 days or less (Connors, Harrison & Akins, 1985). Connors et al. (1985) is the most frequently cited reference in the area of human habitability in the space environment (National Commission on Space, 1986; Oberg & Oberg, 1986). Connors et al. (1985) advocate that steps should be taken to accommodate a wider variety of human needs for long-term human space living. Ride (1987) stated that many crucial issues in the major areas of health, life support, and operational capabilities remain to be resolved before human safety can be assured in the space environment.

Before future plans can be made for space travel, baseline personal hygiene information is needed. The following definitions were determined by the Space Station Personal Hygiene Study (SSPHS) group after extensive review of literature, review by a panel of experts, and contact with various product manufacturers, professional organizations, self-help organizations, and U.S. governmental agencies.

Personal hygiene activities are activities performed to one's own integumentary system (hair, nails, and skin) and oral cavity (mouth) for health maintenance (Czerwinski, 1986) to maintain an individual's operational or functional abilities in a confined environment (NASA, 1987). *Feminine hygiene activities,* the focus of this chapter, are part of personal hygiene activities and include bathing and drying of the entire body, cleansing after defecation/urination, and cleansing the genitourinary area during menses and providing for replacement and disposal of used products (Czerwinski, 1986).

Although women have previously sought astronaut positions in the U.S. space program (Boyle, 1978), the first female crew members were not selected until the late 1970s for the Space Shuttle Program (Brown, 1979). The Space Shuttle Program is an orbiter that takes off as a rocket, orbits as a satellite, and returns to Earth. In June 1983, Sally K. Ride, PhD, became the first American woman in space (Mason, 1983).

Before the selection of the first female astronaut candidates, the first all-female, bed-rest study was conducted in 1973 at the NASA/Ames Human Research facility in California by Sandler and Winter (1978). The 12 volunteer subjects were active Air Force nurses and reservists. The bed-rest period lasted for 17 days, with a 5-day recovery period. The study found that woman are capable of handling weightlessness. According to the authors, "They [women] may be more sensitive subjects for evaluating countermeasures to weightlessness and developing criteria for assessing applicants for Shuttle voyages" (p. 1). The authors also reported that it did not appear that women sent into space will have additional problems because of menstruation. Simulated weightlessness studies of women under the direction of Sandler and Winter have continued into the 1980s (Rowes, 1982), but no discussion of personal hygiene was included.

Baseline information on personal hygiene activities of terrestrial American females is lacking in the research literature on space travel. Information about male personal hygiene activities exists from work done in the early 1970s on flight-experienced males in preparation for Skylab (Fairchild Republic, 1971). During the same time, the Soviets established clothing and personal hygiene requirements from ground-based studies on male subjects (Finogenov, Azhayev, & Kaliberdin, 1973). However, in 1979 Brown suggested a baseline personal hygiene protocol for female spacecraft crew members.

Brown (1979), as part of her work on the anthropometric and physiological differences between males and females, also addressed personal hygiene considerations needed for female crew members to live in space. Brown interviewed the first 21 female candidates for the Astronaut Corps, of which 6 were later selected to be America's first female astronauts. The personal hygiene and related areas addressed in Brown's study were management of menses, shaving leg and underarm hair, and design of waste management facilities including urine collection in the spacesuit. Twenty of the 21 candidates used tampons exclusively and had a preferred brand. This finding was consistent with a larger study conducted by *Consumer Reports* ("Menstrual Tampons," 1978) in which 65% of the women surveyed used tampons.

In considering whether to use tampons in space, the space program has to review an aspect of the tampon that relates to product use and women's health. The use of tampons was regarded as a harmless practice until the Center for Disease Control (CDC) issued warnings identified with the use of tampons as a risk factor in Toxic Shock Syndrome (TSS) (Reame, 1983). Whereas the role of tampons as a cause of TSS is not clear, certain guidelines for use are standard information with tampon packaging (Tambrands, Inc., 1988). Women are advised on the tampon's absorbency and change needs of at least every 6 hours. Handwashing before inserting tampons is recommended. However, there is no information known to the author that demonstrates the women's adherence to these guidelines.

Before further discussing feminine hygiene considerations in space travel, this author asserts certain assumptions. Females are and will continue to be crew members in American space explorations. Menstruation is a normal physiological function, and women have a choice in altering or maintaining this function. Pregnant astronauts will be part of the space station crew (Goldsmith, 1986).

FEMININE HYGIENE CONSIDERATIONS IN SPACE TRAVEL

Three major areas in the application of feminine hygiene need to be considered in space travel. These areas include cleansing of the whole body and the genital-urinary area and collection of menses.

Whole-Body Cleansing

Whole-body cleansing, head to toe, is not available on the Space Shuttle orbiter. Translated, there is no shower facility. Selected partial body cleansing is done by scrubbing with a washcloth, soap, and water. Chemical or "wet" wipes are also available on Shuttle missions for body cleansing.

Proposed for the future Space Station are whole-body cleansing areas, sometimes called "space showers" (Collins, 1988). Because of limited power, water, and space inside the space station, and weight requirements, crew members will most likely be limited to taking a shower every 2 days using 1 gal of recycled water (Czerwinski, 1986). The proposed space station will have a crew of 4–12 people who will live and work in 90-day rotations (Allen & Martin, 1985).

Genital-Urinary Area Cleansing

On the Shuttle, the toilet is called the Waste Management System or space "potty." Designed for both men and women astronauts, the space potty is similar to a toilet with some modifications. These modifications pertain to foot restraints and a seat belt to keep the person using the facility from floating away. The person has to sit in such a way as to obtain a suction between the anal area and the toilet seat to create a vacuum to remove the feces. Likewise, a funnel device (male or female types) is used to pull the urine out of the body (Oberg & Oberg, 1986; Pogue, 1985). On the Shuttle, donning/doffing of clothing by men and women is needed to complete waste management operations.

The Earth's human waste management system, known as the bathroom with a toilet, accommodates all human wastes in one container. A disposal system that would store human wastes compactly and odor-free is under development for the space station (Jennings & Lewis, 1987), because, while in the space environment, humans travel and live within the confines of a closed ecological system until their return to Earth.

Menses Collection

On the Shuttle, tampons and pads are available for female crew members to select for individual personal hygiene kits. Insertion and removal of tampons are done as in the Earth's environment. Waste products from the three female orifices have to be collected separately, packaged, and stored for return to Earth. Men also do the same with their waste products. Considering the limited number of females with flight experiences, the author is unable to find any reference to a crew member having or not having a menstrual cycle while in flight.

FUTURE IDEAS

The following ideas are proposed with a concern for finding answers to further the American space goals.

1 Develop a product or process that would accurately predict the onset of menstruation within 6–12 hr. Menstruation differs from the other eliminative processes, such as urination and defecation, in that there is not a physiological mechanism to allow for voluntary control over the elimination act. The nature of menstruation precludes its being a brief, time-limited phenomenon (Patterson & Hale, 1985). Accurate prediction would enable the crew member to prepare for menstruation by using a menses collection product, such as a tampon or cervical cap, before scheduled activities such as extravehicular activities (EVA) in a spacesuited condition.

2 Develop a cultural variation database related to feminine hygiene practices. This information would be valuable in planning for an international crew on long-duration space flights.

3 Undertake long-term simulation biosphere interdisciplinary studies (Kanas, 1987). These studies could include the use of air-fluidized mattresses to observe physiological changes that people in space might endure.

4 Administer crew acceptance studies to assess individual needs and preferences. Studies can be done by using questionnaires and building mock-up or demonstration personal hygiene facilities layouts and interfaces with other systems for practical experiences and evaluations.

SUMMARY

A basic human need in the space environment will be the ability to maintain health. Space travel in the future will involve large numbers of people living and working together for long periods of time under confined conditions in a hostile environment. Human adjustment will be a key factor to success in space living (Kanas, 1987). One element of human adjustment will be the ability to achieve personal hygiene with limited resources (Brown, 1979; Connors et al., 1985). Questions related to Earth practices for personal hygiene activity of feminine hygiene in space have been partially answered, and research questions and ideas to guide hygiene procedures for space travel planning have been suggested.

REFERENCES

Allen, J. P., & Martin, R. (1985). *Entering space: An astronaut's odyssey.* New York: Stewart, Tabori & Chang, Inc.

Boyle, C. P. (1978, March). Manned and womanned space flight. *Space World, 3,* 22–24.

Brown, J. W. (1979). Considerations associated with the introduction of female crew members in spacecraft and space stations. *Proceedings of the 30th Congress of the International Astronautical Federation.* New York: Pergammon.

Collins, M. (1988). Mission to Mars. *National Geographic, 174,* 733–764.

Connors, M. M., Harrison, A. A., & Akins, F. R. (1985). *Living aloft: Human requirements for extended space-flight.* Washington, DC: Scientific and Technical Information Branch, NASA.

Czerwinski, B. S. (1986). *Unpublished personal diary of the space station personal hygiene study.* Houston: Author.

Fairchild Republic Division, (1971, August 31). *Final report: A baseline protocol for personal hygiene* (Contract NAS 9-11509). Farmingdale, NY: Author.

Finogenov, A. M., Azhayev, A. N., & Kaliberdin, G. V. (1973). Cosmonaut clothing and personal hygiene. *Scientific Translation Service* (NASA-TT-F-14532-Rev.). Washington, DC: NASA.

Goldsmith, M. F. (1986). How will humans act as science fiction becomes fact? *Journal of the American Medical Association, 256,* 2048–2050, 2052.

Jennings, D., & Lewis, T. (1987, May). System for odorless disposal of human waste. *NASA Technical Briefs,* p. 80.

Kanas, N. (1987). Psychological and interpersonal issues in space. *American Journal of Psychiatry, 144,* 703–709.

Mason, R. G. (1983). *Life in space.* Alexandria, VA: Time-Life Books.

Menstrual tampons and pads. (1978, March). *Consumer Reports,* pp. 127–131.

National Aeronautics and Space Administration (NASA). (1987, March). *Man-system integration standards* (NASA-STD-3000; Vols. I, II). Houston, TX: Johnson Space Center.

National Aeronautics and Space Administration (NASA). (1988). *NASA thesaurus: Vol. 1, Hierarchical listing; Vol. 2, Access vocabulary; Vol. 3, Definitions.* Springfield, VA: NASA, Scientific and Technical Information Division.

National Commission on Space, Report of (1986). *Pioneering the space frontier.* New York: Bantam.

Oberg, J. E., & Oberg, A. R. (1986). *Pioneering space.* New York: McGraw-Hill.

Patterson, E. T., & Hale, E. S. (1985). Making sure: Integrating menstrual care practices into activities of daily living. *Advances in Nursing Science, 7*(3), 18–30.

Pogue, W. R. (1985). *How do you go to the bathroom in space?* New York: Tom Doherty Associates.

Reame, N. E. (1983). Menstrual health products, practices, and problems. *Women & Health, 8*(2/3), 37–49.

Ride, S. K. (1987). *Leadership and America's future in space.* Washington, DC: NASA.

Rowes, B. (1982). Housewives in space. *Omni, 4*(4), 64–67, 128.

Sandler, H., & Winter, D. L. (1978). *Physiological responses of women to simulated weightlessness.* Washington, DC: NASA, Scientific and Technical Information Office.

Tambrands, Inc. (1988). *What you should know about toxic-shock syndrome (TSS). Tampax products insert information.* Lake Success, NY: Author.

Chapter 8

The Effect of Premenstrual Symptoms on Creative Thinking

Joan C. Chrisler

INTRODUCTION

Anxiety and depression, in clinical case studies and in experiments unrelated to the menstrual cycle, have been shown to affect cognition (Messick, 1965; Beck, 1976). These findings have led to a number of studies attempting to link cognitive deficits to the premenstrual phase of the menstrual cycle.

Researchers have investigated variations in students' academic performance (Dalton, 1960a, 1960b; Sommer, 1972; Bernstein, 1977; Walsh, Budtz-Olsen, Leader, & Cummins, 1981) and performance on various tests related to academic ability, such as arithmetic (Wickham, 1958; Lazarov, 1982), spelling and vocabulary (Wickham, 1958), anagrams (Golub, 1976; Rodin, 1976), and puzzles (Rodin, 1976).

Studies have been conducted to investigate variations in performance on standardized tests, including Raven's Progressive Matrices (Wickham, 1958), the Watson-Glaser Critical Thinking Appraisal (Sommer, 1972), Hidden Figures (Golub, 1976; Lazarov, 1982), Plot Titles (Golub, 1976), Possible Jobs (Golub, 1976), Digit-Symbol Substitution (Rodin, 1976), the Stroop Color-

Word Interference Test (Rodin, 1976), the Rod and Frame Test (Lazarov, 1982), and the Brief Affect Recognition Test (Lazarov, 1982). None of these studies have reported any significant premenstrual deficits.

Yet the general public, and perhaps the academic community also, continue to believe that such deficits regularly occur. After reviewing a number of studies in this area, Sommer (1973, 1983) concluded that although most objective performance measures fail to demonstrate cycle-related differences, many of the self-report studies indicate impairment, including premenstrual deficits in the ability to concentrate. A recent survey of college students (Golub, 1981) found that 75% of the males and 32% of the females believed that menstruation affects women's thinking processes; 59% of the males and 51% of the females believed that women are less able to function when they are menstruating.

The present study was designed to investigate the following questions: Are there significant menstrual cycle phase differences in the ability to think creatively? Are there significant differences between women's and men's ability to think creatively? Are androgynous subjects more creative than masculine and feminine subjects?

METHOD

Subjects

Twenty women, average age 36.2 years, and 11 men, average age 31.6 years, volunteered to serve as subjects in this study. Most subjects were recruited through signs posted at several small colleges in northern New Jersey. None of the women were using oral contraceptives; all had regular menstrual cycles, with an average length of 28.6 days and a standard deviation of 5.7 days.

Apparatus

Each female subject was given a basal thermometer (model no. SS05; Pymm Thermometer Corporation, Brooklyn, NY) and a graph on which to record her daily temperatures through one menstrual cycle. The subjects received verbal instructions on the use of the thermometer and the graph. Instructions from the company were available in the thermometer box.

Tests and Questionnaires

The Torrance Tests of Creative Thinking (Torrance, 1962) are reliable and valid tests of verbal and figural creative thinking. The verbal tests consist of seven activities: Asking, Guessing Causes, Guessing Consequences, Product Improvement, Unusual Uses, Unusual Questions, and Just Suppose. The figural tests consist of three activities: Picture Completion, Picture Construction, and the Parallel Lines or Circles Task. The tests yield separate scores for fluency (the ability to generate a number of ideas), flexibility (the ability to generate different types of ideas), originality (the ability to generate unique or statistically infrequent ideas), and elaboration (figural tests only: the ability to fill out or elaborate on ideas). Forms A and B, with an average intercorrelation of .88, were administered approximately 15 days apart.

The Bem Sex-Role Inventory (Bem, 1974) consists of 60 adjectives, 20 of which are stereotypically feminine, 20 of which are stereotypically masculine, and 20 of which are neutral filler items without sex-role connotations. Subjects indicate on a seven-point Likert scale how well each item describes themselves. The inventory yields the following classifications: androgynous, feminine, masculine, undifferentiated.

The Menstrual Attitude Questionnaire (Brooks-Gunn & Ruble, 1980) consists of 33 statements that subjects mark, using a seven-point Likert scale, to indicate the strength of their agreement with the attitudes expressed. The statements have been analyzed to yield five attitude factors: menstruation as a debilitating event, menstruation as a bothersome event, menstruation as a natural event, menstruation as an event that can be anticipated and predicted, and denial of the effects of menstruation. Subjects receive a score on each attitude factor; high scores indicate strong agreement.

The Menstrual Distress Questionnaire (Moos, 1968) consists of 47 symptoms or changes in experience that have been associated with the menstrual cycle. Subjects indicate on a six-point Likert scale the extent to which they have experienced each symptom over the course of their last menstrual cycle. The symptoms have been factor-analyzed to yield eight symptom clusters: pain, concentration, behavior change, autonomic reactions, water retention, negative affect, and control. One symptom (change in eating habits) does not fit into any of the clusters. Subjects receive scores for each cluster describing their menstrual, premenstrual, and intermenstrual experiences. High scores indicate strong experience of the symptom cluster.

The subjects were also asked to answer questions about their experience during the testing sessions. They were asked how creative they thought they were, at which testing session they thought they performed better, and what they thought was the aim of the research. Female subjects were asked if they thought the phase of the menstrual cycle generally affected their intellectual or creative performance.

Procedure

The subjects were invited to participate in a study of creativity and biorhythms. They were told that participation would require two 90-min testing sessions and approximately 30 min to fill out miscellaneous questionnaires. Female subjects were also asked to take their temperatures daily for 6 weeks and to record them on a graph.

Testing sessions were arranged for the subjects' convenience, although at-

Table 8-1 Means, Standard Deviations, and *t* Ratios on the Torrance Tests of Creative Thinking for Female (*n* = 20) and Male (*n* = 11) Subjects

Measure	Females	Males	*t*
Verbal combined			
M	209.1	200.7	0.22
SD	73.9	66.0	
Verbal fluency			
M	90.1	87.8	0.16
SD	27.3	27.8	
Verbal flexibility			
M	38.0	38.6	−0.13
SD	8.9	8.9	
Verbal originality			
M	81.0	74.3	0.33
SD	39.4	31.3	
Figural combined			
M	167.0	174.2	−0.28
SD	43.5	50.6	
Figural fluency			
M	20.7	20.5	0.04
SD	6.6	6.1	
Figural flexibility			
M	16.4	16.1	0.12
SD	4.5	3.8	
Figural originality			
M	37.1	31.7	0.78
SD	13.3	11.3	
Figural elaboration			
M	92.8	105.8	−0.62
SD	35.4	42.6	

tempts were made to counterbalance the subjects' exposure to the Torrance Tests. Subjects completed both the verbal and figural forms of the tests at each testing session; the verbal tests were always administered first.

After the second testing session, subjects were given the Bem Sex-Role Inventory, the Menstrual Attitude Questionnaire, and an exit questionnaire that asked about the subjects' beliefs about the experiment. Women were given the Menstrual Distress Questionnaire and asked whether they believed that their menstrual cycle phase affected their intellectual or creative performance.

Postmenstrual testing was carried out on days 7 to 11 and premenstrual testing on days 23 to 27 (or within 5 days of the onset of the menses). Men were tested on the dates of the full moon and the new moon, or within 2 days before or after these dates.

RESULTS AND DISCUSSION

No sex differences in creative thinking were found (Table 8-1). This finding is in agreement with the majority of research (Maccoby & Jacklin, 1974) in this area.

When the data were analyzed by sex-role orientation rather than by sex, androgynous subjects were found to be significantly more creative than feminine subjects as measured by the verbal tests (Table 8-2). It was hypothesized that androgynous subjects, being more flexible and less role-bound, would perform better on the creative thinking tests than either the masculine or the feminine subjects. This hypothesis was only partially supported and only on the verbal tests. Perhaps this results from the fact that the verbal tests require scientific thinking (guessing causes, guessing consequences, hypothesizing) and

Table 8-2 Means, Standard Deviations, and F Ratios on the Torrance Tests of Creative Thinking for Androgynous (n = 9), Feminine (n = 7), Masculine (n = 9), and Undifferentiated (n = 6) Subjects

Measure	And.	Fem.	Masc.	Und.	F
Verbal combined					
M	241.3	166.1	198.2	211.8	3.33[a]
SD	80.2	52.7	62.4	60.7	
Verbal fluency					
M	103.9	73.9	86.8	89.1	3.55[a]
SD	30.3	21.2	25.0	21.7	
Verbal flexibility					
M	42.0	32.5	38.7	38.6	3.13[a]
SD	9.9	5.5	9.2	7.9	
Verbal originality					
M	95.4	59.7	72.7	84.1	2.93[a]
SD	42.7	27.0	30.8	33.0	
Figural combined					
M	184.7	164.8	164.2	160.5	0.91
SD	38.6	53.8	46.1	42.0	
Figural fluency					
M	21.8	20.8	22.2	16.1	2.76
SD	7.7	4.8	5.7	4.9	
Figural flexibility					
M	16.8	15.6	17.9	14.1	2.18
SD	4.9	3.7	4.1	3.0	
Figural originality					
M	37.4	36.4	32.3	34.9	0.51
SD	12.4	14.7	12.2	11.4	
Figural elaboration					
M	108.7	92.0	91.8	95.4	0.72
SD	33.9	41.4	37.1	40.6	

[a]p < .05.

use technical examples (product improvement, finding unusual uses for objects), which may be more familiar to those with masculine sex-role orientations than to those with feminine sex-role orientations.

Data collected on the Menstrual Distress Questionnaire are presented in Table 8-3. These subjects are arithmetically higher on all premenstrual ratings than the younger subjects in Moos' (1977) normative data, which is consistent with the finding that premenstrual symptoms increase with age (Debrovner, 1982). Inspection of the data also indicates that the premenstrual ratings are higher than the menstrual ratings for all scales, suggesting the presence of premenstrual syndrome in this sample. Thus, if premenstrual symptoms are capable of interfering with creative thinking, they should do so in this sample.

Creative thinking scores were analyzed by menstrual cycle phase (Table 8-4), and no significant differences were found. This finding is in agreement with those of other studies (Sommer, 1973) of cognitive abilities, which have reported no significant premenstrual deficits.

Table 8-3   Means and Standard Deviations on the Menstrual Distress Questionnaire for the Menstrual, Premenstrual, and Intermenstrual Phases of the Testing Cycle (*n* = 20)

Scale	M	P	I
Pain			
M	12.9	13.9	8.8
SD	4.7	5.3	3.3
Concentration			
M	10.9	12.8	9.8
SD	2.9	6.2	2.1
Behavior change			
M	7.3	8.0	6.0
SD	2.0	3.1	1.5
Autonomic reactions			
M	4.5	5.2	4.2
SD	0.9	2.5	0.4
Water retention			
M	8.7	12.7	6.7
SD	3.4	3.2	2.9
Negative affect			
M	16.6	23.9	13.6
SD	6.4	9.1	5.7
Arousal			
M	11.2	11.6	11.0
SD	4.3	5.1	4.4
Control			
M	7.6	8.0	7.2
SD	3.3	4.6	2.9

Table 8-4 Means, Standard Deviations, and *t* Ratios on the Torrance Tests of Creative Thinking for the Postmenstrual and Premenstrual Testing Sessions (*n* = 20)

Measure	Postmenstrual	Premenstrual	*t*
Verbal combined			
M	213.2	205.0	0.97
SD	83.2	62.9	
Verbal fluency			
M	91.7	88.6	0.87
SD	30.7	23.4	
Verbal flexibility			
M	38.5	37.5	0.79
SD	9.6	8.2	
Verbal originality			
M	83.0	78.9	0.83
SD	44.4	33.4	
Figural combined			
M	163.7	170.3	−0.96
SD	49.0	36.9	
Figural fluency			
M	20.2	21.1	−0.69
SD	7.5	5.5	
Figural flexibility			
M	16.4	16.5	−0.15
SD	5.1	3.9	
Figural originality			
M	35.8	38.5	−0.78
SD	12.4	14.1	
Figural elaboration			
M	91.4	94.3	−0.60
SD	38.6	31.8	

Thirty-three percent of the women participants expressed the belief that their premenstrual performance was worse than their postmenstrual performance. The scores for these subjects were separated and analyzed (Table 8-5). On the majority of measures calculated, there were no significant differences; however, the women performed significantly better premenstrually on the figural fluency test. Despite their negative expectations, the women performed as well or better than usual.

A separate analysis was also carried out for women who expressed strong negative attitudes toward menstruation (Table 8-6). Again, there were no significant differences in performance on most of the measures of creative thinking. The differences that were found (on the combined figural tests and the figural fluency test) were again in the direction of better performance premenstrually. These findings and those of the previous analysis could be explained by Parlee's

Table 8-5   Means, Standard Deviations, and *t* Ratios on
the Torrance Tests of Creative Thinking for Women
(*n* = 7) Who Believed that Their Performance Would
Show a Premenstrual Deficit

Measure	Postmenstrual	Premenstrual	*t*
Verbal combined			
M	216.1	200.9	0.84
SD	102.0	71.1	
Verbal fluency			
M	90.7	86.7	0.58
SD	34.9	27.4	
Verbal flexibility			
M	37.3	37.4	−0.06
SD	11.1	10.2	
Verbal originality			
M	88.1	76.7	1.03
SD	56.6	34.8	
Figural combined			
M	142.0	152.1	−0.80
SD	41.9	40.9	
Figural fluency			
M	15.3	18.3	−3.33[a]
SD	4.9	5.7	
Figural flexibility			
M	13.9	13.7	0.11
SD	3.8	2.8	
Figural originality			
M	32.7	34.3	−0.22
SD	11.6	14.3	
Figural elaboration			
M	80.1	85.9	−0.55
SD	34.6	31.7	

[a] $p < .05$.

(1983) suggested "premenstrual elation syndrome" or by a determination to work harder to compensate for expected deficits (Rodin, 1976; Bernstein, 1977).

The men's creativity scores were analyzed by moon phase (Table 8-7), and a surprising finding occurred. Although no lunar phase differences were expected, the men performed significantly better on the figural fluency test when the moon was full and significantly better on the figural elaboration test when the moon was new. This is not in agreement with previous research (Rotton & Kelly, 1985), which has generally not found lunar cycle differences despite the general public's belief in them. The present results are probably spurious because of the small number of male participants but may be explained by the fact that subtle cognitive changes have not been studied. Lunar phase research has concentrated on overt behaviors such as accident rates, emergency room visits, psychiatric admissions, and crisis calls.

It is clear that premenstrual changes do not produce cognitive deficits, or, if they do, the deficits are so minor that an extra "push" is all that is needed to compensate. Although the research community has known this for more than a decade, the general public does not. They still hold negative attitudes toward and expectations for premenstrual women, and, no doubt, suspect that instability caused by the menstrual cycle is responsible for women's lesser creative achievements. Any sex differences in creative achievement are far more likely

Table 8-6 Means, Standard Deviations, and *t* Ratios on the Torrance Tests of Creative Thinking for Women (*n* = 13) Who Expressed Negative Attitudes on the Menstrual Attitude Questionnaire

Measure	Postmenstrual	Premenstrual	*t*
Verbal combined			
M	184.4	181.0	0.30
SD	84.8	60.6	
Verbal fluency			
M	80.0	80.9	−0.19
SD	30.2	24.0	
Verbal flexibility			
M	35.0	35.4	−0.31
SD	9.1	8.2	
Verbal originality			
M	69.4	64.7	0.71
SD	46.9	30.6	
Figural combined			
M	144.9	158.2	−1.85[a]
SD	40.4	37.1	
Figural fluency			
M	18.7	20.7	−2.04[a]
SD	6.6	6.0	
Figural flexibility			
M	15.9	16.2	−0.30
SD	4.4	4.4	
Figural originality			
M	31.5	36.1	−1.12
SD	5.5	14.1	
Figural elaboration			
M	78.9	85.2	−1.09
SD	28.5	25.0	

[a]$p < .05.$

Table 8-7 Means, Standard Deviations, and *t* Ratios on the Torrance Tests of Creative Thinking for Men (*n* = 11) at the New Moon and Full Moon Testing Sessions

Measure	New moon	Full moon	*t*
Verbal combined			
M	200.0	201.4	−0.11
SD	72.5	58.9	
Verbal fluency			
M	87.1	88.5	−0.28
SD	32.0	22.9	
Verbal flexibility			
M	37.6	39.7	−0.99
SD	9.2	8.5	
Verbal originality			
M	75.4	73.2	0.38
SD	32.9	29.5	
Figural combined			
M	180.9	167.5	1.67
SD	51.7	48.5	
Figural fluency			
M	19.8	21.2	−0.82
SD	4.8	7.1	
Figural flexibility			
M	15.7	16.6	−2.34[a]
SD	3.3	4.2	
Figural originality			
M	31.5	32.0	−0.14
SD	12.5	9.9	
Figural elaboration			
M	113.9	97.7	−2.89[a]
SD	43.5	40.1	

[a]$p < .05$.

to be caused by lack of opportunities and lack of recognition of women's work than by any biological processes.

REFERENCES

Beck, A. T. (1976). *Cognitive therapy and the emotional disorders.* New York: New American Library.

Bem, S. L. (1974). The measurement of psychological androgyny. *Journal of Consulting and Clinical Psychology, 42*, 155–162.

Bernstein, B. E. (1977). Effects of menstruation on academic performance among college women. *Archives of Sexual Behavior, 6*, 289–296.

Brooks-Gunn, J., & Ruble, D. N. (1980). The menstrual attitude questionnaire. *Psychosomatic Medicine, 42*, 503–512.

Dalton, K. (1960a). Effects of menstruation on schoolgirls' weekly work. *British Medical Journal, 1,* 326–328.

Dalton, K. (1960b). Menstruation and examinations. *British Medical Journal, 2,* 1386–1388.

Debrovner, C. (1982). *Premenstrual tension: An interdisciplinary approach.* New York: Human Sciences Press.

Golub, S. (1976). The effect of premenstrual anxiety and depression on cognitive function. *Journal of Personality and Social Psychology, 34,* 99–104.

Golub, S. (1981). Sex differences in attitudes and beliefs regarding menstruation. In P. Komnenich, M. McSweeney, J. A. Noack, & N. Elder (Eds.), *The menstrual cycle: Research and implications for women's health* (pp. 129–134). New York: Springer.

Lazarov, S. (1982). The menstrual cycle and cognitive function. (Doctoral dissertation, Yeshiva University, 1982). *Dissertation Abstracts International, 43,* 280B.

Maccoby, E. E., & Jacklin, C. N. (1974). *The psychology of sex differences.* Stanford, CA: Stanford University Press.

Messick, S. (1965). The impact of negative affect on cognition and personality. In S. S. Tomkins & C. E. Izard (Eds.), *Affect, cognition, and personality* (pp. 98–128). New York: Springer.

Moos, R. H. (1968). The development of a menstrual distress questionnaire. *Psychosomatic Medicine, 30,* 853–867.

Moos, R. H. (1977). *Menstrual distress questionnaire manual.* Stanford, CA: Stanford University Social Ecology Laboratory.

Parlee, M. B. (1983). Changes in moods and activation levels during the menstrual cycle in experimentally naive subjects. *Psychology of Women Quarterly, 7,* 119–131.

Rodin, J. (1976). Menstruation, reattribution, and competence. *Journal of Personality and Social Psychology, 33,* 345–353.

Rotton, J., & Kelly, I. W. (1985). Much ado about the full moon: A meta-analysis of lunar-lunacy research. *Psychological Bulletin, 97,* 286–306.

Sommer, B. (1972). Menstrual cycle changes and intellectual performance. *Psychosomatic Medicine, 34,* 263–269.

Sommer, B. (1973). The effects of menstruation on cognitive and perceptual-motor behavior: A review. *Psychosomatic Medicine, 35,* 515–534.

Sommer, B. (1983). How does menstruation affect cognitive competence and psychophysiological response? *Women and Health, 8*(2/3), 53–90.

Torrance, E. P. (1962). *Guiding creative talent.* Englewood Cliffs, NJ: Prentice Hall.

Walsh, R. N., Budtz-Olsen, I., Leader, C., & Cummins, R. A. (1981). The menstrual cycle, personality, and academic performance. *Archives of General Psychiatry, 38,* 219–221.

Wickham, M. (1958). The effects of the menstrual cycle on test performance. *British Journal of Psychology, 49,* 34–41.

Part Two

Perimenstrual Symptoms and Perimenstrual Syndromes

Both function and dysfunction have been associated with the menstrual cycle. Although the majority of women experience one or more symptoms around the time of menstruation, they do not experience distress or disability associated with these symptoms. Yet a very few women (probably less than 10% of menstruating women) experience perimenstrual symptoms to such a degree of severity that it would be considered a syndrome. In this section, the distinction between perimenstrual symptoms and perimenstrual syndromes is explored, and methodological issues, explanatory mechanisms, and treatment protocols are proposed. In addition to the discussion of perimenstrual symptoms and syndromes, women's health problems that vary with the menstrual cycle are investigated.

Delineation and precise measurement of perimenstrual symptom patterns remain a challenge to researchers in this field. Mitchell, Woods and Lentz (Chapter 9) report on the methodology used to define perimenstrual symptom severity patterns. Using criteria developed from a population-based sample, 27 distinct symptom severity patterns were identified. Only two of the symptom patterns were similar to the premenstrual syndrome (PMS) symptom pattern, raising questions about the accuracy of diagnosis of the PMS symptom pattern in clinical practice and the homogeneity of the samples of previous studies of PMS.

Many investigators, in attempts to delineate diagnostic syndromes, have reported that negative affect symptoms, anxiety, rapid mood changes, and psychophysiological arousal emerge as the prominent factors accounting for much of the distress experienced by women in the perimenstruum. To understand the multiple factors involved in the experience of perimenstrual negative affect, Taylor, Woods, Lentz, Mitchell and Lee (Chapter 10) applied computerized structural equation modeling strategies (LISREL VI) to a large, randomly selected, multiethnic database. The most prominent finding from this causal analysis was that women who had stressful lives and who were generally distressed had the most severe perimenstrual negative affect. Moreover, the effect of stressors not only was direct, but operated through generalized distress (anxiety and depression unrelated to menstrual cycle phase).

Methodological and clinical questions arise about whether perimenstrual symptoms (particularly the negative affect symptom cluster) represent menstrual cycle variations in psychological stress, manifestations of chronic stress, or a frank psychiatric disorder. To understand these differences, Chuong, Colligan, Coulam and Bergstralh (Chapter 11) evaluated the psychological status of 20 women with PMS and 20 women without PMS using the Minnesota Multiphasic Personality Inventory (MMPI). Their results show that women with PMS had many statistically and clinically significant changes in MMPI response patterns throughout their cycles. These authors also support the evidence for PMS subgroups. They found one group with significant changes during the cycle and a smaller group with significant psychological dysfunction throughout the cycle. These two groups may represent perimenstrual magnification of underlying negative affectivity or a psychiatric disorder.

Research directed to clinical therapeutics for perimenstrual symptoms and syndromes continues as a focus for a number of investigators. Robertson (Chapter 12), in a survey of 40 PMS centers in the United States, found that the majority of treatments for PMS include interdisciplinary and multidimensional approaches. Whereas dietary treatments were recommended by most health care providers (92%), hormone treatments were recommended 80% of the time, psychological counseling was recommended over half of the time, and in 20% of the PMS centers, intervention was directed to the children of the women experiencing PMS.

Miota, Yahle and Bartz (Chapter 13) report on the experience of the PMS Treatment Program at the Milwaukee Psychiatric Hospital. These authors are therapists and describe the philosophy of the PMS Treatment Program, which defines premenstrual symptoms as adaptive—allowing women to use the monthly emotional and behavioral changes for personal growth. Data are presented on 66 of the women in the treatment program with one third of the women in an inpatient psychiatric setting and over 70% of the women reporting a family history of substance abuse.

Menstrual dysfunction may include phenomena other than PMS. Hapidou and DeCatanzaro (Chapter 14) report on a study of pain sensitivity in dysmenorrheic and nondysmenorrheic women as a function of menstrual cycle phase. This carefully designed study improved on previous studies by incorporating multiple dependent measures of pain assessment (pain tolerance, subjective pain ratings, pain threshold) and testing two opposing models of pain (adaptation-levels model, hypervigilance model). Although the two groups differed significantly in their ratings of menstrual pain, no significant difference was found between the dysmenorrheic and nondysmenorrheic women on any of the pain ratings at any of the menstrual cycle phases.

Although headache is a frequent complaint associated with the menstrual cycle, little research has been done examining the differences in menstrually related headaches and those occurring at other times. Solbach, Coyne and Sargent (Chapter 15) in a study of headache intensity and disability across the menstrual cycle found that although menstrually related headaches appeared different than those occurring at different times, there were no significant differences between the two types of headaches. The mean ratings of intensity and disability were relatively low for the menstrually related headaches suggesting that although women are aware of the headache, they continue to pursue activities.

Finally, Coughlin (Chapter 16) reports on the correlation between diagnosed breast disease and multiple health-related variables including menstrual cycle factors. Although previous research indicates that prolonged menstrual activity associated with early menarche and later menopause increases the risk for developing breast cancer, this association was not proved in this study even when statistical correction included the number of births. The author suggests that more normal values for some breast disease tests may be found in the follicular phase of the menstrual cycle and after some dietary and lifestyle modifications. The author recommends client education concerning the best time for breast self-examination and breast screening procedures.

Chapter 9

Recognizing PMS When You See It: Criteria for PMS Sample Selection

Ellen S. Mitchell, Nancy F. Woods, and Martha J. Lentz

INTRODUCTION

Premenstrual syndrome (PMS) was first described in 1931 (Frank, 1931). The most common definitions of PMS are based on the timing of symptoms in terms of both amount and direction of change in severity across the menstrual cycle. A typical definition is a group of symptoms that reoccur cyclically, increase in severity just before menses (premenses), abate sometime after the onset of menses, remain low in the postmenses phase, and interfere in some way with daily living (Halbreich, Endicott, & Lesser, 1985; Rubinow & Roy-Byrne, 1984). However, symptoms that vary in severity in a cyclical pattern in a menstruating woman do not always indicate that PMS is present. Missing in most definitions of PMS, and in most sampling procedures for PMS studies, are specific severity level criteria that define low severity postmenses and high severity premenses, specific criteria for an adequate amount of change in severity between postmenses and premenses, and a standardized procedure for distinguishing the PMS symptom pattern from other cyclically reoccurring severity patterns that may be present. In other words, to define an adequate change in severity across the cycle and to distinguish one severity pattern from another, a standard list of symptoms and cut-off criteria that represent minimum and maximum severity levels are needed to define low, medium, and high severity (Mitchell, Lentz, Woods, Lee, & Taylor, in press).

As studies of PMS proliferate, more homogeneous samples are needed for greater precision in detecting group differences and differences across the menstrual cycle. Precision in identifying a PMS sample is important to avoid a heterogeneous mix of symptomatic women with problems other than PMS causing their symptoms. It is possible that earlier PMS treatment studies that revealed no group differences between women with PMS and those with low symptoms failed to detect real differences that might have been present but were attenuated because of heterogeneous samples. Also, PMS studies that have demonstrated group differences or differences across the menstrual cycle may not actually reflect differences in women with PMS but some other condition inadvertently represented in the sample. To advance our knowledge about causes of PMS, to enhance our ability to conduct clinical trials, and to help clinicians diagnose and treat women with PMS, it is imperative that efforts be made to define this symptom pattern more specifically. Currently, the PMS symptom pattern is not always recognized when present or is thought to be present when it is not.

Retrospective reports of PMS without prospective documentation are unreliable. Over half of women who volunteer to take part in PMS studies do not have PMS when their symptom-severity patterns are evaluated prospectively by daily rating forms (Rubinow, Roy-Byrne, Hoban, Gold, & Post, 1984). In one study, when the prevalence of retrospective reports of 47 different perimenstrual symptoms was compared with prospective reports of the same symptoms, almost all of the 47 symptoms were reported by 4% to 53% more women using the recall approach than with the daily approach (Woods, Most, & Dery, 1982). These findings reflect the existence of stereotypical bias in symptom reporting, leading to overreporting of symptoms at premenses when they are expected to occur (Ruble, 1977).

Another pitfall in the identification of women with PMS is to focus on symptom severity only during the premenstrual phase of the menstrual cycle. Just because a woman reports high-symptom severity premenstrually does not necessarily mean she has PMS. High premenstrual symptom severity could reflect chronic symptom distress, that is, consistently high severity throughout the menstrual cycle, or it could reflect the premenstrual exacerbation of symptoms that exist throughout the rest of the cycle, that is, high symptoms postmenses and even higher premenses. This pattern of premenstrual symptoms exacerbation is called premenstrual magnification (PMM) (Harrison, 1982) and represents another form or pattern of cyclically reoccurring symptoms that can interfere with daily living. Therefore, whenever PMS sampling occurs it is important that a consistent method be used to differentiate between PMS and PMM severity patterns.

Work by Rubinow, Roy-Byrne, Hoban, Gold, and Post (1984) reflects an attempt to improve the precision of a PMS definition by requiring a prospective daily rating of negative mood symptoms for three menstrual cycles, with at least a 30% increase in symptom severity from the postmenses week to the premenses week in two of the three cycles. This more recent refinement is a beginning step in the quest for more precision with PMS sample selection. It establishes measurable criteria for a minimal amount of change in severity across the menstrual cycle. However, it is unclear from the literature how the 30% change figure was derived. Also, using only a percentage change in severity does not account for a baseline minimum (floor) or maximum (ceiling) severity level against which the percentage of change is measured. This lack of a standardized base could result in a PMS sample that includes women with a wide diversity of absolute change in symptom severity across the cycle. Without criterion-based severity levels women could be included in a PMS sample who have a 30% change in severity but have a very small absolute change. For example, a postmenses severity score of 4 and a premenses score of 5.2 would indicate a 30% change that may be barely perceptible. In the same sample a woman could also be included with a fairly high postmenses score of 18 and a high premenses score of 23.4, which also represents a 30% change. These two examples both meet the 30% change criterion but represent two different symptom severity patterns. The first example is a consistently low severity pattern, whereas the second is more likely either PMM or a chronically high symptom-severity pattern.

Neither of these situations reflects the classical PMS pattern (low severity postmenses and high severity premenses). Therefore, the key issue for identifying women with PMS pattern, and for differentiating the PMS pattern from the PMM pattern or other perimenstrual symptom patterns, is the establishment of maximum severity levels for the definition of low severity postmenses and premenses (ceiling) and minimum severity levels for the definition of high severity postmenses and premenses (floor), in addition to the development of criteria defining an adequate amount of change.

The purposes of this study were: (1) to describe the process of development, in a normative sample, of cut-off criteria reflecting the *combination* of severity level and amount of change in severity across the menstrual cycle to identify different symptom-severity patterns in menstruating women; (2) to differentiate the PMS and PMM symptom-severity patterns from each other; and (3) to describe the prevalence of the resulting symptom-severity patterns in a population-based sample. The aim of this work is to promote consistency and homogeneity in sample selection across studies about menstrual cycle symptom severity by developing a method other investigators and clinicians can use reliably.

DEVELOPMENT OF THE CRITERIA

Sampling

The community-based, cross-sectional sample on which this method was based was obtained through a multistage sampling procedure. Street segments were identified and randomly ordered by computer from census block groups selected according to age, income, ethnicity, and educational criteria to reflect the general population of a large northwestern metropolitan city. Telephone numbers were obtained from a city directory for households within the street segments. Contact was made with 5,755 households by telephone, and 1,135 women between the ages of 18 and 45 years were identified. From this pool of potential participants, 656 women were eligible and completed an in-home interview and were given instructions about how to keep a daily health diary. Women with complete diary data for at least one full menstrual cycle (a total of 327 women) comprised the sample for development of the cut-off criteria. Inclusion criteria included an age between 18 and 45 years old, not currently pregnant, not being treated for a gynecological problem, having menstrual periods, and having the ability to write and understand English. Women taking birth control pills were included in the sample.

Sample Characteristics

The women in this sample of 327 generally were employed (76%) and married or partnered (61%). Sixty-six percent were Caucasian, 16% Black, and 15% Asian. The average number of years of education was 14.3 years, the mean family income was between $29,000 and $30,999, and the women had a mean age of 32.4 years (SD = 6.8). Fourteen percent (n = 45) were taking birth control pills, and 66% had been pregnant at least once. The mean cycle length was 29.5 days (SD = 5.3), and mean menses length was 5.3 days (SD = 1.7).

Procedure

The process of development of the cut-off criteria for forming symptom-severity subgroups involved six steps: (1) designing an initial symptom list for daily data collection, (2) collecting symptom severity level data daily from a large, community-based population of menstruating women, (3) determining the specific daily symptoms to score, the specific days of the cycle to label as the postmenses and premenses days, and the number of days to score, (4) scoring daily symptoms for all diaries for symptom severity using the selected symptoms and specified postmenses and premenses days, (5) calculating a total group mean score and standard deviation for postmenses and premenses, plus a mean difference score (postmenses score minus premenses score) and standard deviation, and (6) forming symptom severity subgroups based on the derived criteria.

Symptom Selection The initial symptom list was part of the original Washington Women's Health Diary (WWHD), developed by our research team, and included a list of 57 negative and positive symptoms frequently reported to change across the menstrual cycle (Woods, Lentz, Mitchell, Lee, & Taylor, 1986; Woods, 1987). The 57 symptoms were derived from several menstrual symptom questionnaires, including the Moos Menstrual Distress Questionnaire (Moos, 1968), the Premenstrual Assessment Form (Halbreich, Endicott, Schach, & Nee, 1982), and the Rating Scale for Premenstrual Tension Syndrome (Steiner, Haskett, & Carroll, 1980). Items were selected to include those most frequently associated with the perimenstruum. Some of the items from the questionnaires were rephrased to make them more specific (i.e., insomnia became three items: difficulty in getting to sleep, awakening during the night, and early morning awakening; change in eating became four items: increased and decreased appetite and increased and decreased food intake).

Eligible women in the community who agreed to participate were instructed by a trained interviewer about how to keep the diary. Each day the 57 symptoms in the WWHD were rated on a scale from 0 (not present) to 4 (extreme). The women were asked to complete the diary for three menstrual cycles. Symptoms from the first complete cycle of data were used for the development of the cut-off criteria. A complete cycle was defined as one with a clear-cut start and end of the menstrual cycle, plus at least 3 days of available data in the designated postmenses and premenses days for all symptoms scored.

A factor analysis was performed on the 57 symptoms in the WWHD. First, items were removed if they had minimal variance or if they were redundant based on intercorrelations of .80 or higher. A principal component analysis with an orthogonal rotation was then done on the remaining items, which provided a final six-factor solution. Five of the factors contained negative symptoms, whereas one factor contained mostly positive experiences. All final factors had an eigenvalue of 1.0 or more and had factor loadings of .40 or more. Thirty-three symptoms were then selected as the basis for the scoring procedure based on two criteria: (1) the symptom had to be negative or distressful since that is the typical PMS presentation, and (2) the symptom had to be in one of the five negative symptom clusters from the factor analysis. These 33 symptoms were labeled the Menstrual Symptom Severity List-Daily (MSSL-D) (Table 9-1).

Defining Postmenses and Premenses Days For symptom-severity scoring, postmenses was defined as days 4 to 10, with day 1 the first day of menses. Premenses was defined as days -7 to -1, that is, the 7 days before the next menses. The postmenses days were selected to avoid the typically symptomatic menses days and to represent a time of relatively low estrogen level and before the rapid rise in estrogen in the late follicular phase (Speroff, Glass, & Kase, 1983). The premenses days were selected because they represented the most frequently reported days of symptom reporting in the PMS literature. Data from

Table 9-1   The Menstrual Symptom Severity List (MSSL-D) Embedded in the Original Symptom List of the Washington Women's Health Diary

Daily Experience List

Please read the list of feelings and behaviors. Please fill in the blank next to the number that best describes how you felt today. Fill in 0 for each day if not present.

0	1	2	3	4
Not present	minimal	mild	moderate	extreme

1. * Abdominal pain, discomfort	_____	30. * Hostility	_____
2. * Anger	_____	31. * Hot flashes or sweats	_____
3. * Anxiety	_____	32. * Impatient, intolerant	_____
4. * Awakening during the night	_____	33. Impulsiveness	_____
5. * Backache	_____	34. In control	_____
6. * Bloating or swelling of abdomen	_____	35. Increased activity	_____
7. Blurred or fuzzy vision	_____	36. Increased appetite	_____
8. Bursts of energy of activity	_____	37. Increased food intake	_____
9. Confusion	_____	38. * Increased sensitivity to cold	_____
10. Cramps-uterine or pelvic	_____	39. Increased sexual desire	_____
11. * Craving for specific foods or tastes	_____	40. * Increased sleeping	_____
12. Craving for alcohol	_____	41. Intentional self-injury	_____
13. Decreased appetite	_____	42. * Irritable	_____
14. * Decreased food intake	_____	43. * Lonely	_____
15. * Decreased sexual desire	_____	44. Lowered coordination/clumsiness	_____
16. * Depression (feel sad or blue)	_____	30. * Lowered desire to talk/move	_____
17. * Desire to be alone	_____	46. Nausea	_____
18. Diarrhea	_____	47. Nervousness	_____
19. * Difficulty concentrating	_____	48. * Out of control	_____
20. * Difficulty in getting to sleep	_____	49. * Painful or tender breasts	_____
21. * Difficulty making decisions	_____	50. * Rapid mood changes	_____
22. Dizziness or lightheadedness	_____	51. Restlessness or jitteriness	_____
23. * Early morning awakening	_____	52. * Sensation of weight gain	_____
24. Fatigue or tiredness	_____	53. * Skin disorders	_____
25. * Feelings of guilt	_____	54. Suicidal ideas or thoughts	_____
26. Feelings of well-being	_____	55. * Swelling of hands or feet	_____
27. Forgetfulness	_____	56. * Tearfulness, crying easily	_____
28. General aches and pains	_____	57. * Tension	_____
29. * Headache	_____		

*The 33 symptoms used to create severity level and cycle phase difference criteria.
Copyright © 1990 by N. F. Woods, E. S. Mitchell, and M. J. Lentz. Not to be reproduced in whole or part by any process without written permission from the authors.

the postmenses and premenses days within the same menstrual cycle were used to examine symptom responses to the same ovarian follicle and set of physiological events.

    Selection of Days to Score   To obtain mean symptom severity scores for postmenses and premenses, calculations were initially performed based on a method described by Abraham (1983) in which scores for 7 days postmenses and 7 days premenses were totaled for the 33 critical symptoms. The worst 3 days of the 7 were then selected, and a mean score for these worst 3 days was calculated. However, this method had an increased chance of error because it required handscoring, and since it reflected the pattern of severity for only 3 of the 7 days of interest, the approach was changed to include the mean of all 7 postmenses and premenses days as the basis for the symptom-severity scores. By using all 7 days in the calculations, the severity scores would more closely reflect the 7-day symptom-severity pattern reported in the diary and could be scored by computer to reduce error.

Refinement of Days to Score The next step in the refinement process was to reduce the number of days scored in the postmenses and premenses from 7 to 5 days. This was done to narrow the slice of time sampled to increase the chances of sampling days that were more physiologically similar. For post-menses, days 6–10 were selected for scoring and, for premenses, days -5 to -1. This approach also avoided menstrual flow days for the postmenses phase (mean number of menses days was 5.3 in this normative sample), avoided days -6 to -8 when estrogen and progesterone levels peak (Speroff et al., 1983), and more closely reflected the time when ovarian hormone levels were drop-ping premenses.

Calculation of Severity Level Criteria A 5-day group mean and stan-dard deviation (SD) ($N = 327$) were calculated for postmenses and premenses severity using the individual mean scores for the 5 postmenses and 5 premenses days. Once the population-based sample mean and SD were obtained, three levels of severity were identified for both postmenses and premenses: low, medium, and high severity (Table 9-2). A medium severity level was created by spreading the upper limits of low severity and the lower limits of high severity by 1/2 SD. This was done by adding 1/4 SD to the group mean score and subtracting 1/4 SD from the group mean score (mean $\pm$ 1/4 SD). The forma-

Table 9-2 Symptom Severity and Cycle Phase Difference (CPD) Criteria for Classifying Menstrual Cycle Symptom Severity Patterns

	Postmenses[a] criteria	Premenses[b] criteria	CPD[c] criteria Level	CPD[c] criteria Score
High severity	≥ 10.5	≥ 12.1	Large	≥ 6.2
Medium severity	6.6–10.4	7.8–12.0	Moderate	3.7–6.1
Low severity	≤ 6.5	≤ 7.7	Small	≤ 3.6

[a]Postmenses 5-day group mean = 8.53, SD = 7.97.
[b]Premenses 5-day group mean = 9.96, SD = 8.67.
[c]Cycle phase difference group mean = 4.92, SD = 5.19.

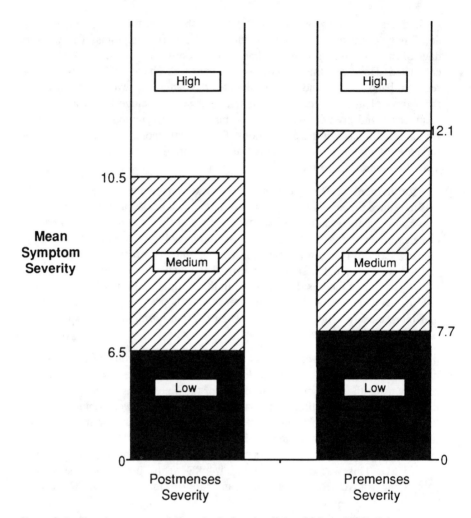

Figure 9-1   Five-day mean severity criteria for classifying 33-item MSSL-D into symptom severity patterns.

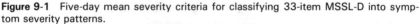

tion of the medium severity level using the 1/2 SD spread created mutually exclusive categories (low, medium, high) with consistently detectable differences, without being so restrictive that membership in the high and low severity groups would be difficult to obtain. Using this 5-day mean ± -1/4 SD approach, three levels of severity were calculated for postmenses and three levels for premenses. The low severity criterion for postmenses had a lower limit of 0 and a maximum level of 6.5, which was 1/4 SD below the group postmenses mean (M = 8.53, SD = 7.97) (Figure 9-1). The high severity criterion had an infinitely high maximum level and a minimum level of 10.5, which was 1/4 SD

above the group postmenses mean (Figure 9-1). The resulting postmenses medium severity criterion was a score greater than 6.5 and less than 10.5. The
three levels of severity computed for premenses (M = 9.96, SD 8.67) were a
low severity criterion of 0 to 7.7, a high severity criterion of 12.1 or higher,
and a medium severity criterion of 7.8 to 12.0 (Figure 9-1).

Calculation of Change in Severity To define an adequate amount of
change in severity across the menstrual cycle with enough power to achieve
consistently detectable differences in severity, a difference score called a cycle
phase difference (CPD) was calculated by subtracting the mean severity score
for postmenses from the mean severity score for premenses for each woman
and then obtaining the population-based sample mean and SD for these difference scores (M = 4.92, SD = 5.19). Three mutually exclusive levels of cycle
phase difference were calculated (small, moderate, and large difference), using
the 1/2 SD-minimum spread criterion to form the moderate difference level
(Table 9-2). Again the moderate level was formed by adding and subtracting 1/4
SD to and from the sample mean (mean ± 1/4 SD) to ensure the ability to
detect a moderate difference in severity from postmenses to premenses. These
calculations resulted in a small CPD criterion from 0 to 3.6, a large CPD
criterion of 6.2 or greater, and a moderate CPD criterion between 3.7 and 6.1
(Figure 9-2). These three groups of criteria (the postmenses and premenses
severity criteria and the CPD criteria) were then used to classify each woman in
the sample into a symptom severity pattern.

Creating Symptom Severity Subgroups When the postmenses and premenses severity level criteria were applied to the severity scores for each
woman in the sample, it was possible to classify each woman into 1 of 9
symptom patterns based on low, medium, and high severity postmenses and/or
premenses, for example, low severity postmenses and high severity premenses
(LH), high severity postmenses and medium severity premenses (HM), or high
severity postmenses and even higher severity premenses (HH) (Table 9-3).
When the three CPD criteria were added to the classification of the nine possible severity level patterns, there were 27 different symptom-severity patterns
available for classification. For example, a severity pattern of low severity
postmenses (L) and high severity premenses (H) could have a small, moderate,
or large CPD (LH/S, LH/M, or LH/L), or a severity pattern of high severity
postmenses (H) and premenses (H) could have a small, moderate, or large CPD
(HH/S, HH/M, HH/L). In addition, if direction of change in severity across the
cycle were included in the classification, each of the subgroups could be further
broken down. For practical purposes, because the focus of this study was on the
PMS and PMM symptom patterns, only the high severity subgroups (HH) were
further classified by direction of change. This resulted in six subgroups with
high severity postmenses and high severity premenses; three of the subgroups
were increasing and three were decreasing in severity across the cycle. When

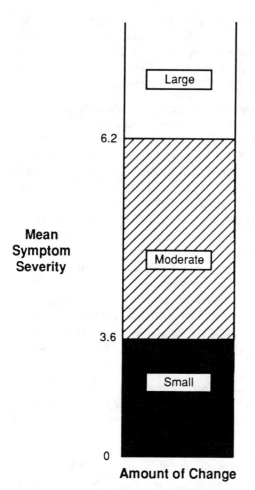

Figure 9-2 Criteria for classifying 33-item MSSL-D into amount of change in severity across the menstrual cycle (postmenses to premenses).

all the women in the sample ($N = 327$) were classified using the severity level, the CPD criteria, and direction of change, they fit into 21 different symptom severity patterns (Table 9-3). Six patterns had no cases represented (LL/L, LH/S, LH/M, MM/M, MM/L, HL/S).

Defining PMS and PMM Using the severity level, CPD, and direction of change criteria (Table 9-2), it was then possible to identify a woman with a PMS symptom pattern (i.e., low symptoms postmenses and an adequate increase premenstrually). The women in the sample were classified into a PMS symptom pattern if they had either the low postmenses/high premenses/large CPD pattern (LH/L) or the low postmenses/medium premenses/large CPD pattern (LM/L). In other words, all women who had low postmenses symptom severity for the 33-symptom MSSL (a mean score of 6.5 or less for days 6 to 10), had either medium severity (a mean score of 7.8 to 12.0) or high severity (a mean score of 12.1 or more) premenses (days -5 to -1), and had a large difference in severity from postmenses to premenses (6.2 or more) were identified as having a PMS symptom pattern (Table 9-4).

The inclusion of both the LH and LM severity patterns in the PMS sample creates the possibility of a very small difference in severity between postmenses (≤ 6.50) and premenses (≥ 7.8) if *only* severity level were considered. However, by requiring the additional CPD criterion, at least a 6.2-point spread in severity from postmenses to premenses must exist to say that an adequate increase in severity occurred. For example, if the postmenses severity were 6.5, the required 6.2 CPD would represent more than a 100% change in severity. Thus, to be classified in the PMS symptom pattern, if a postmenses score was 6.5 then the minimal premenses score must be 12.7, a 6.2 difference. Likewise, if the postmenses score was 0, the lowest acceptable premenses score for the PMS symptom pattern would be 7.8.

Women with a PMM pattern similarly were identified as those with a large CPD (a 6.2 or more difference), symptom severity that increased across the

Table 9-3 Prevalence of Symptom-Severity Patterns in a Population-Based Sample (N = 327) using 5-Day Mean Scores for Postmenses and Premenses

[a]SS pattern		Cycle phase difference		
[b]Post	Pre	Small	Moderate	Large
[c]L	L	111 (34.0%)	11 (3.4%)	0
L	M	3 (1.0%)	15 (4.6%)	[e]9 (2.7%)
L	H	0	0	[e]23 (7.0%)
M	L	15 (4.6%)	3 (1.0%)	3 (1.0%)
M	M	20 (6.1%)	0	0
M	H	1 (0.3%)	4 (1.2%)	[f]10 (3.0%)
H	L	0	3 (1.0%)	8 (2.4%)
H	M	11 (3.4%)	5 (1.5%)	9 (2.7%)
H	H			
	[d]inc.	10 (3.0%)	11 (3.4%)	[f]18 (5.5%)
	dec.	9 (2.7%)	7 (2.0%)	8 (2.4%)

[a]Symptom severity pattern.
[b]Post, postmenses severity level; Pre, premenses severity level.
[c]L, low severity; M, medium severity; H, high severity.
[d]inc., severity increasing across the cycle for HH; dec., severity decreasing across the cycle for HH.
[e]Part of PMS symptom pattern.
[f]Part of PMM symptom pattern.

Table 9-4   PMS[a] and PMM[b] Symptom-Severity Pattern Criteria

	Postmenses criteria	Premenses criteria	CPD[c] criteria
PMS	≤ 6.5	≥ 7.8	≥ 6.2
PMM	≥ 6.6	≥ 12.1	≥ 6.2

[a]PMS, low postmenses severity + medium or high premenses severity + large CPD.
[b]PMM, medium or high postmenses severity + high premenses severity + large CPD.
[c]CPD, cycle phase difference.

cycle, a medium or high severity score postmenses (a mean score of 6.6 or more), and a high severity score premenses (12.1 or more) (HH/L or MH/L) (Table 9-4). Women with this PMM symptom pattern were symptomatic in both cycle phases but had a definite increase (≥ 6.2) in severity across the cycle. Thus, by using this criterion-based method to classify the sample into specific symptom severity patterns, the PMS and PMM patterns were clearly delineated and differentiated from each other. This resulted in distinctly different and homogeneous symptom patterns.

PREVALENCE OF SYMPTOM SEVERITY SUBGROUPS

When the prevalence of each of the 27 possible severity patterns and the PMS and PMM symptom patterns was examined, the largest subgroup was the one with consistently low symptom severity and small CPD (LL/S), representing 34% (n = 111) of the sample (Table 9-3). When all the women with increasing symptom severity and a large CPD were grouped together (LM/L, LH/L, MH/L, HH/L), they represented 18.3% (n = 60) of the sample (Table 9-3). When the sample was divided into the PMS and PMM symptom patterns, 9.8% (n = 32) of the sample demonstrated the PMS pattern and 8.6% (n = 28), the PMM pattern. Women with a large CPD that decreased across the cycle represented another 28 (8.6%) of the sample (ML/L, HL/L, HM/L, HH/L), and those with consistently high symptom-severity postmenses and high severity premenses with a small CPD (HH/S) consisted of 19 (5.8%) of the population-based sample. Finally, it was of interest to determine if birth control pills had any effect on the group means used to create the criteria. When women on birth control pills (n = 45) were compared with those taking no hormones (n = 282), there were no differences for postmenses or premenses mean severity scores or for the CPD mean score.

SUMMARY

The focus of this study was the development of criteria for the identification of distinct menstrual cycle symptom severity patterns in menstruating women. Using criteria developed from a population-based sample, 27 distinct symptom-severity patterns were identified. This ability to classify the symptom experiences of menstruating women into many different severity patterns, with only two comprising the PMS symptom pattern, raises questions about the homogeneity of the samples of previous PMS studies and the accuracy of the diagnosis of the PMS symptom pattern in clinical practice. It is likely that women with symptom patterns other than PMS were included in many PMS studies in the past. It is also likely that clinicians used PMS intervention strategies with women who were thought to have the PMS pattern but who really had a different symptom pattern. The use of a criterion-based classification system derived from a population-based sample presented in this paper is one means by which investigators designing future PMS studies could select more homogeneous samples, reduce misclassification bias, enhance statistical power, and obtain more consistent results across studies.

Finally, these findings have implications for health care providers who care for women with PMS. The existence of many severity patterns other than the PMS pattern points to the need for a careful evaluation of the specific symptom pattern presented by each woman before a diagnosis is made and definitive therapy is begun. Use of a daily symptom record in clinical practice, which includes the 33-symptom MSSL-D plus the application of the cut-off criteria for scoring symptom severity and determining CPD, could help clinicians in their diagnostic evaluation of women who present with distressful symptoms that reoccur cyclically. With a more precise diagnosis, clinicians could then target their therapy more appropriately.

REFERENCES

Abraham, G. E. (1983). Nutritional factors in the etiology of the premenstrual tension syndromes. *The Journal of Reproductive Medicine, 28,* 446–464.

Frank, R. T. (1931). The hormonal causes of premenstrual tension. *Archives of Neurology and Psychiatry, 26,* 1053–1057.

Halbreich, U., Endicott, J., & Lesser, J. (1985). The clinical diagnoses and classification of premenstrual changes. *Canadian Journal of Psychiatry, 30,* 489–497.

Halbreich, U., Endicott, J., Schach, S., & Nee, J. (1982). The diversity of premenstrual changes as reflected in the premenstrual assessment form. *Acta Psychiatrica Scandinavica, 65,* 46–65.

Harrison, M. (1982). *Self-help for premenstrual syndrome.* New York: Random House.

Mitchell, E. S., Lentz, M., Woods, N. F., Lee, K., & Taylor, D. (in press). Methodologic issues in the definition of premenstrual symptoms. In A. J. Dan & L. L. Lewis

(Eds.), *Menstrual health in women's lives: Proceedings of the 1985 research conference of the Society for Menstrual Cycle Research.* Chicago: University of Illinois Press.

Moos, R. (1968). The development of a menstrual distress questionnaire. *Psychosomatic Medicine, 30,* 853–867.

Rubinow, D. R., & Roy-Byrne, P. (1984). Premenstrual syndromes: Overview from a methodologic perspective. *The American Journal of Psychiatry, 141,* 163–172.

Rubinow, D. R., Roy-Byrne, P., Hoban, M. C., Gold, P. W., & Post, R. M. (1984). Prospective assessment of menstrually related mood disorders. *American Journal of Psychiatry, 141,* 684–686.

Ruble, D. (1977). Premenstrual symptoms: A reinterpretation. *Science, 197,* 291–292.

Speroff, L., Glass, R. H., & Kase, N. G. (1983). *Regulation of the menstrual cycle in clinical gynecologic endocrinology and infertility* (3rd ed.) (pp. 75–83). Baltimore/London: Williams & Wilkins.

Steiner, M., Haskett, R. F., & Carroll, B. J. (1980). Premenstrual tension syndrome: The development of research diagnostic criteria and new rating scales. *Acta Psychiatrica Scandinavica, 62,* 177–190.

Woods, N. F. (1987). Premenstrual symptoms: Another look. *Public Health Reports Supplement,* July/August, 106–107.

Woods, N. F., Lentz, M., Mitchell, E., Lee, K., & Taylor, D. (1986). *Prevalence of perimenstrual symptoms* (Final Report NU 1054). Division of Nursing, USPHS, Washington, D.C.

Woods, N. F., Most, A., & Dery, G. K. (1982). Estimating perimenstrual distress: A comparison of two methods. *Research in Nursing and Health, 5,* 81–91.

Chapter 10

Perimenstrual Negative Affect: Development and Testing of an Explanatory Model

Diana Taylor, Nancy F. Woods, Martha J. Lentz, Ellen S. Mitchell, and Kathryn A. Lee

INTRODUCTION

In the clinical sciences, we are confronted with an accumulating mass of clinical and experimental data, gathered by many different (and often conflicting) methodologies and based on limited theoretical premises that do not consider the complexity of human health phenomena. Historically, practice theories and models provided an all-encompassing explanation unsupported by empirical evidence. Alternately, clinical research unguided by theory has created data resulting from sophisticated research methodologies but remains unorganized, incoherent, or interpretively constrained to the limits of a narrow population sample or its own conceptual paradigm. With the advances made in computer-assisted structural equation modeling, it is now possible to build and test complex theoretical models using multidimensional data found in the clinical environment.

This research was supported in part by a grant, Prevalence of Perimenstrual Symptoms (NU1054), from the Division of Nursing, USPHS.

This study extended a theory of perimenstrual symptom experience (Woods, Most, & Dery, 1982; Woods, 1985) by applying structural equation modeling strategies, specifically linear structural relationships (LISREL VI). Specifically, structural equation models were used to systematically extend and test a theoretical model that explains the antecedents and consequences of women's perimenstrual symptom experience. The original theory (Woods, Dery, & Most, 1982; Woods, 1985b) is a multidimensional theory of perimenstrual symptom experience, which includes the concepts of perimenstrual symptom perception, the influence of socialization experiences, the social environment, health status, health practices, perception of stress, and menstrual cycle characteristics.

A refined theoretical model was first developed using the confirmatory factor analysis function of the LISREL VI computer program, and the complete LISREL solution was applied to test the theoretical model. LISREL is both a general mathematical model and a computer program for the analysis of covariance structures (Joreskog & Sorbom, 1985). Data from one subsample of women ($n = 222$) were used for theory refinement, and another subsample of women were used for theory testing ($n = 119$). These theoretical models were fitted to a multiple indicator database collected on a multiethnic random sample of nonpatient women ($N = 656$).

The Conceptual Model: Antecedents of Perimenstrual Symptom Experience

Popularly referred to as premenstrual syndrome (PMS), various symptoms associated with the perimenstruum have a major impact on women's health regardless of the lack of agreement as to its cause, definition, significance, and management (Clare, 1985; Abplanalp, 1983; Reid, 1986; O'Brien, 1987; Brown & Harrison, 1986). Recent studies suggest that a cluster of symptoms that include negative affect, low impulse control, cognitive change, and psychophysical arousal may account for much of the distress experienced by women in the perimenstruum (before and during menstruation) (Moos, 1968; Abraham, 1980; Endicott & Halbreich, 1982; Woods, Lentz, Mitchell, Lee, & Taylor, 1987; Taylor, 1986, 1988). To distinguish this symptom cluster from a defined syndrome, the label perimenstrual negative affect (PNA) will be used in the following explanatory model.

Most etiological studies emphasize either a single biological or behavioral explanation for PNA and have not differentiated symptomatic women according to specific types of symptoms or severity levels of symptoms. Because menstrual function is associated with ovarian activity, most researchers have focused on the biological etiologies with little attention to psychosocial or environmental variables. A few investigators have suggested that socialization in a traditional feminine role may be linked to menstrual symptoms (Paige, 1973).

Moreover, expectations and attitudes about menstruation may socialize a woman to experience (PNA (Brooks-Gunn, Ruble, & Clarke, 1977).

There is also evidence for differential effects of stressors on perimenstrual symptoms, with the major effect seen on negative affect (Woods, 1985). The effect of stress may be additive by enhancing the negative perception of perimenstrual symptoms, or the stress response may provide a direct effect by disrupting the hypothalamic-pituitary-ovarian axis. To date, mediating variables such as personality, health status, health behaviors, or socioeconomic status have not been considered in any explanatory model of PMS or PNA. Woods's theory suggests that a woman's perimenstrual symptom experience is multidimensional and occurs in a personal and social context. Any explanatory model must incorporate personal and social variables in addition to physical ones into a biopsychosocial etiology of PNA.

Theoretical Hypotheses and Causal Linkages

Theoretical modeling combined with research evidence taken from our previous factor analytic and reliability studies suggest some causal linkages among antecedent variables in the development of PNA. In particular,

1 Women exposed to many life stressors will experience more distress, perform fewer health promotion practices, and have more severe PNA than their counterparts.
2 Women with more years of education will experience less distress, perform more health promotion practices, and experience less severe PNA than their counterparts.
3 Women socialized in a traditional feminine role will experience more distress, perform fewer health promotion practices, and experience more severe PNA than their counterparts.
4 Women socialized to negative expectations of menstruation experience more distress, perform fewer health promotion practices, and experience more severe PNA than their counterparts.
5 Women experiencing distress (depression/anxiety) will experience severe PNA.
6 Women who perform more health promotion practices will experience less severe PNA.

See Figure 10-1 for a visual description of the proposed theoretical relationships.

METHODS

Data Collection and Population Sampling

To test these hypotheses, data were collected on a randomly selected sample of 656 nonpatient women in a large urban community of the northwestern United

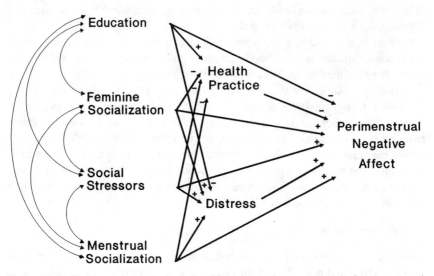

Figure 10-1 Proposed theoretical relationships: An explanatory model of perimenstrual negative affect (PNA).

States. The sampling framework employed in this study involved multiple steps. Census block groups (fractions of census tracts) meeting a particular income criterion ($12,900–$39,000) were sorted to identify those in which 10% or more of the population were Black or Asian. The most suitable block groups from the standpoint of age, ethnicity, and educational groups were identified by the research team. The street segments of the selected census block groups were then identified and randomly ordered with a computer program. The numbers of the street segments within block groups provided the link between this initial set of criteria and a city directory of all addresses in Seattle, from which the sampling units (telephone numbers of all potential participants) were chosen. Contact with 5,755 of the sampling units was completed. Information on the characteristics of the unit was obtained in 4,847 (84%) of the contacts. From this pool of potential subjects, 656 women completed interviews, a conservative response rate of 58%.

This approach generated a population-based sample of women consisting of 103 Asians, 149 Blacks, 374 Whites, and 30 Native Americans, Hispanics, and others. The women ranged in age from 18 to 45, with a mean age of 32.7 years. They reported a mean educational level of 14.2 years and mean income range from $29,000–$30,999. In this group of women 75.9% reported some level of employment outside the home. Currently 57.7% were married or partnered; 27.2% had never married, and 14.4% were divorced or separated. From this group of 656 women, two subsamples were chosen for model development and testing. The first subsample consisted of the first 222 women who completed daily health diaries (and symptom recordings) for at least one menstrual cycle and who demonstrated marked cycle phase differences in symptom severity. The second subsample consisted of 119 women who had regular menstrual cycles, were not using oral contraception, and reported modest cycle phase differences and moderate symptom severity levels.

Design

The hybrid design involved cross-sectional, prospective, and retrospective elements. After households were screened to identify eligible women willing to participate in the study, participants completed an in-home interview and a 90-day health diary. After women completed their diaries, some were asked to participate in a food diary component of the study. Following completion of the 90-day diary and/or the food diary, all women completed a telephone interview. Data reported here are drawn from the initial interview (socialization, stress, distress, education, menstrual cycle characteristics, and health practices) and the daily diary (PNA and health practices).

Concepts and Measured Indicators

Table 10-1 includes the theoretical dimensions (latent concepts), measured indicators, measurement model parameters (reliability estimates), and structural equation parameter estimates. Each of the theoretical dimensions and their measured indicators will be discussed.

Perception of PNA Symptoms In the context of women's perimenstrual symptom experience, women appraise or perceive their bodily sensations, noting certain types of symptoms, feelings, and cognitions that are different from the usual or functional daily experience. Symptom perception is followed by symptom evaluation with factors such as severity, frequency, duration, and visibility influencing how the woman defines the symptoms on the health-illness continuum. The meanings attached to symptoms are useful for understanding and predicting the individual's symptom response, which may include defining symptoms as an illness, taking action through self-care activities, or obtaining professional treatment.

The measurement of symptom perception in this study refers to the participants' ratings of the presence and intensity of symptoms obtained day-by-day from a 90-day health diary. The symptom checklist of the daily diary includes 57 items rated on a 0 (not present) to 4 (extreme) scale. The items included in the health diary were generated from several sources, including the Moos Menstrual Distress Questionnaire (Moos, 1968), Halbreich and Endicott's Premenstrual Assessment Form (Halbreich, Endicott, Schach, & Nee, 1982), work by Woods, Most, and Dery (1982), and other literature.

The latent variable or concept, PNA, was reflected in three symptom clusters obtained by principal component factor analysis (Lentz, Woods, & Mitch-

Table 10-1   Model Development: Measurement Model of Perimenstrual Negative Affect (PNA) LISREL VI Maximum Likelihood Estimates (n = 222)

Dimensions	Abbreviation	Indicator(s)	Measurement model loadings	LISREL model loadings
Education	EDUC	Years of education	.90	.90
		(Mother's symptoms)	(.42)[a]	
Feminine socialization	FEMSOC	Attitudes toward women scale	.99[b]	.88
		Familism scale	.68	.76
		(Denial of symptoms)	(.28)[c]	
Menstrual socialization	MENSSOC	Negative effects of menstruation/premenarcheal preparation	.75	.82
		Mother's symptoms	.42	.43
		Denial of symptoms	.40	.43
Social stressors	STRESS	Life events scale	.90	.90
Health practices	HP	Health practices index	.90	.90
Distress	DIS	CESD depression scale	.93	.92
		Lewis anxiety scale	.83	.79
Perimenstrual	PNA	Premenstrual turmoil	.61	.52
		Menstrual turmoil	.80	.89
		Menstrual out of sorts	.67	.75

[a]Menstrual socialization and education share "mother's symptoms" as an indicator.
[b]The indicator "attitudes toward women scale" and "negative effects of menstruation were specified to share error variance.
[c]Feminine socialization and menstrual socialization share denial of symptoms as an indicator.

ell, submitted). Premenstrual "turmoil" (consisting of hostility, tension, anger, anxiety, mood swings, irritability, guilt, impatience, depression, feeling out of control, tearfulness, for days -1, -3, and -5), menstrual "turmoil" (consisting of depression, tearfulness, anger, anxiety, loneliness, guilt, tension, difficulty making decisions, nervousness, restless, nausea, for days 1, 3, and 5), and menstrual "feeling out of sorts" (consisting of impatience, lowered desire to talk, irritability, out of control, for days 1, 3, and 5) comprised the indicators of PNA.

Gender-Specific Socialization Experiences   Conceptually defined as "socialization to the feminine role" and "socialization specific to menstruation," gender-specific socialization was measured by several indicators. Indicators of feminine socialization included the Attitudes Toward Women Scale (ATW, Spence & Helmreich, 1978) and the familism scale (Paige, 1973). General attitudes toward women were measured with the ATW, a 15-item scale containing statements that describe the roles, rights, and privileges women should have. A 4-point scale is used, ranging from "agree strongly" to "disagree strongly." Items are scored 0–3, with high scores indicating a pro-feminist, egalitarian attitude. Possible total scores range from 0–45. Internal consistency was high (Cronbach's alpha = .86) in this current study sample (Spence & Helmreich, 1978). Familism, valuing the family's well-being over the individual woman's well-being, was measured using the 7-item scale developed by Paige (1973). A 4-point scale is used with high scores on the familism scale indicating that the woman does not agree that the family's well-being should take precedence over her own.

The influence of gender-related events on feminine socialization was conceptualized as the effects of menarche and menstruation on the female enculturation process. Menstrual socialization includes the attitudes, beliefs, expectations, and evaluation of menarche (first menstruation) and menstruation (cyclical recurrence of menses). Indicators of this socialization process included denial of the effects of menstruation (Brooks-Gunn et al., 1977), menstrual symptoms expectancies (Brooks-Gunn & Ruble, 1980), and mother's perimenstrual symptom experience. The Menstrual Attitude Questionnaire by Brooks-Gunn and Ruble (1980) is a 5-scale instrument (33 items) that taps five dimensions of menstrual attitudes: menstruation is a debilitating event, a bothersome event, or a natural event; anticipation and prediction of the onset of menstruation; and denial of any effect of menstruation. Women rate each item on a 7-point scale such that 1 = disagree strongly and 7 = strongly agree. Scale homogeneity was high in previous studies (Cronbach's alpha = .80 − .93). The denial subscale created the strongest factor in the development of our measurement model using confirmatory factor analysis. Menstrual expectations learned before menarche were assessed by asking women to rate 12 items they had been told to anticipate with menstruation (e.g., feeling crabby or irritable). Women also rated their recollections of their mother's experience of 13 different perimenstrual symptoms.

Perception of Stress In this model, a woman's social environment provides both stressful and challenging life events, and supportive or nonsupportive social relations. Originally conceptualized as an accumulation of life strains, the concept of life stress has come to include the qualitative and perceptual nature of the stressor, implying that a stressful social milieu, as perceived negatively by the individual, can be associated with illness (Sarason, Siegel, & Johnson, 1978). Using this expanded definition in our current model, the negative perception of stress was associated with health/illness outcomes such as perimenstrual symptom experience. Furthermore, Woods (1985) adds a contextual dimension by suggesting that a woman's perception of negative life events is embedded within the context of the menstrual experience or the socialization to feminine role and gender-specific events.

The strongest indicator of life-stress perception was the negative life events scale of the Sarason Life Events Survey (LES) as modified by Norbeck (1984). The 91-item LES describes events related to health, work, school, residence, love and marriage, family and close friends, personal and social, financial, crime and legal matters, and parenting. Norbeck (1984) modified the LES to increase the relevancy to women's lives by adding items related to fertility control, finding a job versus home, and being assaulted. Each item requires three responses: event occurrence in the past year, perception of event as good or bad, and magnitude of effect rated as 0 for no effect to 3 for great effect.

Socioeconomic/Educational Status Socioeconomic status (SES) is traditionally conceptualized by multiple dimensions of income, occupation, education, and parents' occupation(s) and income. Using income and occupation to rate a woman's SES, results are often confusing and uninterpretable when entered into a causal structural equation because of the confounding factors of gender-related social inequities and the inverse relationship of education and women's occupation. Thus, education becomes a more precise and discriminating indicator of SES than multiple indicators. Occupation correlated moderately well with education in the initial reliability studies. However, due to the lack of interval-level data and restricted variance in the occupation variable, occupation was deleted as an indicator of SES. In this model, years of education were a reliable indicator of women's social status.

Health Practices Good health practices have been shown to have a cumulative effect on health independent of age, sex, and economic status. In this model, health practices serve as a mediating variable in the severity and perception of perimenstrual symptoms. Dimensions of health-related behaviors include sleep, diet, exercise, and self-care activities. Health-related practices were assessed using a modification of the Human Population Laboratory Questionnaire (Belloc & Breslow, 1972). These questions examine personal habits related to cigarette smoking, use of alcoholic beverages, sleeping habits, physical recreational activities, and nutrition as measured by regularity of meals and weight in relation to height. Participants were asked specific items about their usual hours of sleep; how often they ate breakfast; how often they ate between meals; their weight and height; and physical activity including active sports, swimming or taking long walks, working in the garden, and the like.

Because of the cumulative effect of health practices, a weighted scale was calculated and was called the Health Practices Index (Lentz, 1986). The Health Practices Index includes the variables of hours of sleep, how often the women ate breakfast, incidence of between-meal snacking, weight, height, physical activity and exercise, frequency and duration of cigarette use, and frequency and duration of alcohol use. High scores indicated high levels of healthy behaviors.

Distress Persistent, or noncyclical, negative affectivity was considered a intrapersonal variable influencing the severity and perception of PNA. Conceptualized as a combination of depression and anxiety, negative affectivity results in a personal feeling of distress for the individual woman. In this model, distress was a mediating dimension along with health practices affecting the perception and severity of perimenstrual symptoms. Two indicators, depression and anxiety, represent this latent variable. Depression was measured with the Center for Epidemiologic Studies-Depression Scale (DES-D), designed for use with community populations. In the 20-item scale, respondents are asked how often the symptoms occurred during the past week, and responses are scored on a scale of 0 to 3, where 0 = less than 1 day, and 3 = 5–7 days. A single summarized score is generated with those below 16, indicating the absence of depression. The scale correctly identified 71% of minor depressives, clinically diagnosed patients, and 57% of depressive personalities. The CES-D has a false positive rate of 16.6% and a false negative rate of 40% for major depression. Selected sample means include 3.6 for working women and 4.5 for homemakers (Newberry, Weissman, & Myers, 1979). Reliability of the CES-D in our previous studies was high (alpha = .89). Anxiety was assessed using a 5-item scale (Lewis, Firsich, & Parsell, 1979) scored similarly to the CES-D.

ANALYSIS

A causal model of perimenstrual symptom experience had been conceptualized before the analysis. The raw data generated by the measured indicators were summarized in two forms, a correlation and a covariance matrix. Both matrices were used to develop the measurement model in a confirmatory factor analysis of LISREL VI (Joreskog & Sorbom, 1985) computer program. The measurement model was developed using data from 222 women who completed daily health diaries for at least one complete menstrual cycle and who demonstrated significant cycle phase differences in symptom severity. The respecified model was subsequently tested with data from a different sample of 119 women who exhibited only modest cycle phase differences and had only moderate symptom severity levels. No model respecification occurred during the model testing phase.

The Mathematical Model

The path diagram in Figure 10-1 graphically displays the hypothesized patterns of causal relations among the set of latent variables (unobserved concepts) and the measured variables (indicators). Single-headed arrows represent the direct causal effect of one variable on another. Curved double-headed arrows indicate that two variables are correlated. The model attempts to account for variation and covariation in the "endogenous" variable (PNA) by specifying its causal dependence on other endogenous variables or mediating variables (health practices, distress) and on "exogenous" causal variables (socialization, education, stress).

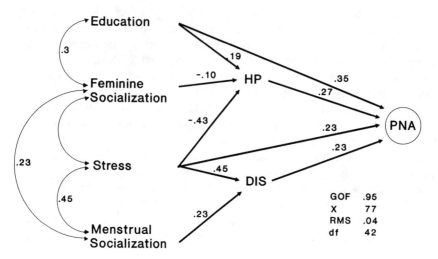

Figure 10-2   PNA theory development: Final structural equation model (n = 222).

Model Development

The Measurement Model   The measurement model specifies how the hypothetical constructs (latent variables) are measured in terms of observed indicator variables. It also describes the measurement properties (e.g., correlations,
covariances) of the measured indicators. Table 10-1 describes the final measurement model and standardized covariance estimates for the theory development
phase. The equations of the measurement component closely resemble a basic
factor-analytical model and can be viewed as confirmatory factor analyses,
where the measured indicators have been specified a priori to have nonzero
loadings on the latent unmeasured concepts. The benefit of this process is that
the measurement error can be accounted for via the examination of large error
terms resulting from the confirmatory factor analysis. The theoretical model
can be respecified using a combination of theory-based and LISREL solutions,
such as removing indicators with large error terms or by allowing latent variables to "share" indicators.

The Structural Equation Model   The structural equation component of
the mathematical LISREL model refers to the hypothesized causal relationship
among the latent variables or abstract theoretical constructs. The objective of
LISREL is to reproduce the observed covariance matrix as closely as possible
and to determine the goodness-of-fit of the model to the data (Herting, 1985).
Unlike path analysis, LISREL uses a maximum likelihood estimation procedure
that estimates all parameters simultaneously. Figure 10-2 describes the final
stage of development of a causal model of PNA.

Three statistics were used in comparing the developing models of PNA: the goodness-of-fit index (GOF), the chi-square statistic (x^2), and the root mean square residual error (RMS). These measures of overall fit between the observed and the predicted models for the three structures compared in the model development phase can be found in Figure 10-2.

Model Testing

During theory development using LISREL, respecification of relationships between latent variables and their measured indicators and respecification of causal relationships is considered procedurally appropriate. However, once the best fit has been achieved between the observed and predicted models and then tested against a new population sample, further respecification can be likened to multiple testing in a traditional hypothesis testing situation. To avoid this problem, we developed the theoretical model using one sample of women ($n = 222$) from the original sample of 656 women. The final respecified model was tested on a different sample of 119 women to further confirm the reliability and validity of the proposed theory. Figure 10-3 graphically describes this model along with the path estimates and overall measures of fit statistics.

RESULTS

Measurement Model: Theory Development

Multiple indicators of latent variables were included for the concepts of "socialization to the feminine role," "distress," "socialization to menstruation," and "perimenstrual negative affect." For the constructs "education/SES," "perception of life-stress," and "health practices," single indicators were used

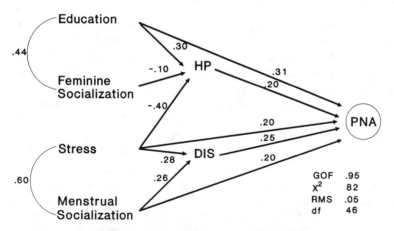

Figure 10-3 PNA theory testing: final structural equation model ($n = 119$). A test of the perimenstrual negative affect theory: A structural equation model using LISREL VI.

because of the high initial reliability estimates. With low measurement error variance, the parameter estimates for these indicators can be constrained at a .90 coefficient level. Model modifications included removing a weak indicator of menstrual socialization and removing self-esteem as an indicator of distress. Further respecification included the allowance of shared error variance between the indicator "attitudes toward women scale" (FEMSOC) and the indicator "negative effects of menstruation" (MENSOC) and allowing two pairs of latent concepts to share indicators (symptom denial: FEMSOC + MENSOC; mother's symptoms: EDUC + MENSOC).

Structural Equation Model: Theory Development

The causal relationship were estimated using the maximum likelihood estimation procedures of LISREL applied to the final measurement model. Further respecification of the causal models resulted in removal of the construct "menstrual socialization," which markedly improved the GOF parameters but was unsupported by theory. Reentering "menstrual socialization" in the theoretical model provided a balance between structural and theoretical soundness. Although self-esteem remained a strong indicator, it was highly correlated with both endogenous and exogenous concepts and created an unstable overall model. Because of the constraints of LISREL, an indicator with multiple correlations among exogenous and endogenous variables must be removed to fit an overall model. The final theoretical model of PNA (Figure 10-2) provided the best fit between the predicted theoretical model and the observed database model as demonstrated in a high GOF index (.95), a significantly low χ^2 (77, d.f. 42, $p < .01$), and a RMS error variance near to zero (.04).

Structural Equation Model: Theory Testing

Only minor differences were found in comparing the two causal models of PNA (development subsample, testing subsample). The final explanatory model (Figure 10-3) derived from subsample no. 2 ($n = 119$) closely replicated that for subsample no. 1 ($n = 222$). The results from this structural equation model analysis showed that women with the most severe social stressors ($r = .28$) and the most negative menstrual socialization ($r = .26$) experienced the most distress. Women with the most severe social stressors also reported the fewest health practices ($r = -.40$), but women with the most education reported the greatest number of health practices. Feminine socialization had a negligible effect on health practices ($r = -.10$). Together, education, health practices, stress, distress, and menstrual socialization influenced PNA. Education was positively associated with PNA ($r = .31$) as were health practices ($r = .20$). Women who experienced the most stressors ($r = .20$), the most distress ($r = .25$), and the most negative menstrual socialization ($r = .20$) experienced the most severe PNA.

DISCUSSION

In general, a theoretical development and testing procedure using structural equations and maximum likelihood estimation (LISREL) supported a theory of PNA. Theory was described, modeled, specified, and tested using concept analysis, confirmatory factor analysis, and LISREL procedures. Data from one subsample of women were used for the model development procedures, and another subsample of women was chosen for the model testing procedures. Because the two subsamples were not randomly selected from the larger sample ($N = 656$), systematic differences were suspected. However, the major causal relationships among latent variables were similar between the two samples.

The most prominent finding in both models (Figures 10-2 and 10-3) is that women who had stressful lives and who were generally distressed had the most severe PNA. Moreover, the effect of stressors was not only direct, but operated through generalized distress (anxiety and depression unrelated to menstrual cycle phase). These findings are consistent with our earlier studies and those of others (Wilcoxon, Schrader, & Sherif, 1976; Siegel, Johnson, & Sarason, 1979; Woods, 1985; Woods et al., 1987; Mills, 1989; Taylor, 1988). Perception of stress appears to increase perimenstrual symptom severity, and negative affect symptoms are more related to reported stress than somatic symptoms. Women who were the most stressed performed few health practices; however, women's health promotion/prevention patterns appeared to do little to alleviate PNA.

Socialization to negative expectations of menstruation also influenced PNA directly, but more clearly through general distress. These results encourage explanation of how exposure to a symptomatic mother and negative messages about menstruation affect mental health and health behavior. Perhaps these indicators reflect socialization processes that indirectly influence negative affect through mother's dysphoria.

That women with more education had more severe symptoms was surprising, but it may be a function of their socialization to health and symptom-reporting. Well-educated women are likely to be more knowledgeable about their health and have the ability to describe their symptom experiences to a greater degree than women who have less education. Description of negative affectivity may be more common among well-educated women compared to the description of physical symptoms. Moreover, well-educated women may be more likely to have expanded expectations for women that have not been met with support from society.

Although socialization to a feminine role appeared to perform weakly in the causal structure, this variable was moderately correlated with two other exogenous variables, education and menstrual socialization. Future analysis may demonstrate that attitudes, social status, and gender-related socialization events are multiple components of a larger construct of feminine socialization.

The finding that women who are generally distressed also have PNA may reflect some women's experience of negative affectivity, a disposition to experience adverse emotional states. Individuals with high negative affectivity tend to be distressed and have a negative view of themselves. Individuals with negative affectivity report nervousness, tension, worry, anger, scorn, revulsion, guilt, self-dissatisfaction, sense of rejection, and sadness. Individuals with negative affectivity are likely to feel negative at all times and in different situations, regardless of overt stress. Moreover, individuals with high negativity are especially sensitive to minor failures, frustrations, and limitations of daily life (Watson & Clark, 1984). It is possible that negative affectivity may mediate the effects of a stressful life on PNA for some women. This explanation would account for the relationship observed between depression and anxiety and perimenstrual symptoms in other studies (Clare, 1983).

Whether negative affectivity is learned is unclear. The finding that socialization to negative expectations of menstruation (including teaching about menstruation and exposure to a symptomatic mother) were related to general distress may reflect one process by which negative affectivity is acquired. Exposure to negative images about being a woman from maternal symptom experience and menstrual teachings may contribute to development of a negative way of viewing the world as well as oneself.

It is of interest that socialization to negative expectations about menstruation did not influence PNA directly, but instead was related to general distress. The positive relationship of negative expectations about menarche to health behaviors underscores the separateness of negative affectivity and behavior. Perhaps women who observed their mothers' symptom experiences become conscious of the need to prevent illness and promote their own health.

This explanatory model of perimenstrual symptom experience includes personal, environmental, and biopsychosocial factors. PNA appears to be a different experience than somatic perimenstrual symptoms. Focusing on only the biological explanations for symptoms, such as ovarian steroid and neurotransmitter models of perimenstrual symptoms, is likely to be of limited utility in understanding women's experiences of PNA. Women with PNA differ from others not only in their symptom patterns, but also in their socialization patterns and general level of distress. Women with PNA symptoms are generally distressed and live difficult lives, but are well educated. These findings underscore the need for a holistic understanding of women's symptom experiences embedded within the broader social issues that affect their lives.

REFERENCES

Abplanalp, J. (1983). Psychologic components of the premenstrual syndrome: Evaluating the research and choosing the treatment. *Journal of Reproductive Medicine, 28,* 517.

Abraham, G. (1980). Premenstrual tension. *Current Problems in Obstetrics and Gynecology, 3,* 7–12.

Anderson, J. G. (1987). Structural equation models in the social and behavioral sciences: Model building. *Child Development, 58,* 49–64.

Belloc, N., & Breslow, L. (1972). Relationship of physical health status and health practices. *Preventive Medicine, 1,* 409–421.

Brooks-Gunn, J., & Ruble, D. (1980). The menstrual attitude questionnaire. *Psychosomatic Medicine, 42,* 503–512.

Brooks-Gunn, J., Ruble, D., & Clarke, A. (1977). College women's attitudes and expectations concerning menstrual related changes. *Psychosomatic Medicine, 39,* 288–298.

Brown, M. A., & Harrison, S. (1986). A comparative analysis of stress in women with varying levels of premenstrual symptomatology. *Communicating Nursing Research, 19,* 15.

Dillon, W., & Goldstein, M. (1988). Linear structural relations (LISREL). In W. Dillon & M. Goldstein (Eds.), *Multivariate analysis: Methods and applications.* New York: John Wiley & Sons.

Clare, A. (1983). Psychiatric and social aspects of premenstrual complaint [Monograph]. *Psychologic Medicine Suppl. 4,* 3–58.

Clare, A. (1985). Psychiatric and social aspects of premenstrual complaint. [Monograph]. *Psychologic Medicine, 4,* 3–58.

Endicott, J., & Halbreich, U. (1982). Psychobiology of premenstrual change. *Psychopharmacology Bulletin, 18*(3) 109–113.

Halbreich, U., Endicott, J., Schach, S., & Nee, J. (1982). The diversity of premenstrual changes as reflected in the premenstrual assessment form. *Acta Psychiatrica Scandinavica, 62,* 177–180.

Herting, J. (1985). Multiple indicator models using LISREL. In H. Blalock (Ed.), *Causal models in the social sciences.* New York: Aldine.

Joreskog, K., & Sorbom, D. (1985). *LISREL VI: Analysis of linear structural relationships by the method of maximum likelihood (3rd ed.).* Mooresville, IN: Scientific Software.

Lentz, M. (1986). The health practices index. *Final report: Prevalence of perimenstrual symptoms.* USPHS, NU1054. Seattle, WA: University of Washington.

Lentz, M., Woods, N., & Mitchell, E. (submitted). Factor structure for daily symptom reports.

Lewis, F., Firsich, S., & Parsell, S. (1979, April). Clinical tool development for adult chemotherapy patients: Process and content. *Cancer Nursing, 2*(2) 99–106.

Mills, (1989). The impact of stress on PMS severity for women in couple relationships. *Proceedings of the Society for Menstrual Cycle Research.* Salt Lake City, UT: University of Utah.

Moos, R. (1968). The development of a menstrual distress questionnaire. *Psychosomatic Medicine, 48,* 388–414.

Newberry, P., Weissman, M. M., & Myers, J. K. (1979). Working wives and housewives: Do they differ in mental states and social adjustment? *American Journal of Orthopsychiatry, 49,* 282–291.

Norbeck, J. (1984). Modification of life event questionnaires for use with female respondents. *Research in Nursing and Health, 7,* 61–71.

O'Brien, P. (1987). Controversies in premenstrual syndrome: Etiology and treatment. In B. E. Ginsburg & B. F. Carter (Eds.), *Premenstrual syndrome.* New York: Plenum Press.

Paige, K. (1973). Women learn to sing the menstrual blues. *Psychology Today, 7,* 41–46.

Reid, R. (1986). Premenstrual syndrome: A time for introspection. *American Journal of Obstetrics and Gynecology, 155*(5), 921–926.

Sarason, R., Siegel, J., & Johnson, J. (1978). Assessing the impact of life changes: Development of the life experiences survey. *Journal of Consulting and Clinical Psychology, 46,* 932–946.

Siegel, J., Johnson, J., & Sarason, I. (1979). Life changes and menstrual discomfort. *Journal of Human Stress, 5,* 41–56.

Spence, J., & Helmreich, R. (1978). *Masculinity and femininity: Their psychological dimensions, correlates, and antecedents.* Austin: University of Texas Press.

Taylor, D. (1986). Development of perimenstrual symptom typologies. *Communicating Nursing Research, 18,* 25.

Taylor, D. (1988). *Nursing interventions for perimenstrual turmoil: A longitudinal therapeutic trial.* Unpublished dissertation. Seattle, WA: University of Washington.

Watson, D., & Clark, L. A. (1984). Negative affectivity: The disposition to experience aversive emotional states. *Psychological Bulletin, 96,* 465–490.

Wilcoxon, L., Schrader, S., & Sherif, C. (1976). Daily self reports on activities, life events, moods and somatic changes during the menstrual cycle. *Psychosomatic Medicine, 38,* 399–417.

Woods, N. (1985). Relationship of socialization and stress to perimenstrual symptoms, disability, and menstrual attitudes. *Nursing Research, 34,* 145–149.

Woods, N., Dery, G., & Most, A. (1982). Estimating the prevalence of perimenstrual symptoms. *American Journal of Public Health, 72,* 1257–1264.

Woods, N., Most, A., & Dery, G. (1982). Toward a construct of perimenstrual symptoms. *Research in Nursing and Health, 5,* 123–136.

Woods, N., Lentz, M., Mitchell, E., Lee, K., & Taylor, D. (1987). Premenstrual symptoms: Another look. *Public Health Reports Suppl.,* pp. 106–112.

Chapter 11

The MMPI as an Aid in Evaluating Patients with Premenstrual Syndrome

C. James Chuong, Robert C. Colligan,
Carolyn B. Coulam, and Erik J. Bergstralh

INTRODUCTION

Since Frank (1931) first described cyclic changes occurring before menses, premenstrual syndrome (PMS) has been viewed as a complex of symptoms characterized by psychologic changes that include irritability, aggressiveness, tension, anxiety, and depression, and by somatic changes, such as feeling bloated, weight increase, edema, breast tenderness, and headaches, all attributed to fluid retention. Part of the differential diagnosis requires that this broad collection of symptoms also be evaluated in terms of mental health status—namely, do the symptoms represent menstrual cycle variations in psychologic stress or are they manifestations of chronic stress or a frank psychiatric disorder?

To assess these potentially cyclical changes in psychologic status, the Min-

The authors thank Gretchen I. Steinmetz, RN, for her assistance.

Reprinted with permission from Chuong, C. J., Colligan, R. C., Coulam, C. B., & Bergstralh, E. J. (1988). The MMPI as an aid in evaluating patients with premenstrual syndrome. *Psychosomatics, 29,* 197–202.

nesota Multiphasic Personality Inventory (MMPI) was administered during the follicular and luteal phases of the menstrual cycle to 20 women with PMS and 20 women without PMS.

SUBJECT SELECTION PROCEDURES

Twenty patients coming for evaluation of menstrual-cycle problems who met the PMS diagnostic criteria to be described agreed to participate in the study. The mean duration of symptoms in the PMS study group was 68.1 months. Twenty female volunteers from among the employees at the Mayo Clinic served as the control group. They had regular, predictable menses and claimed no premenstrual symptoms.

Participants were 18 to 49 years old with regular menses for six or more prior cycles. All were in good health and had normal serum levels of glucose, prolactin, and total thyroxine. By means of a daily diary, each patient reported at least three of the following symptoms (including one or more somatic and psychologic symptoms) within the last half of the cycle for three or more preceding menstrual cycles: irritability, tension or anxiety, mood swings or emotional lability, restlessness, decreased concentration, depression, aggression, poor coordination, cravings for sweet or salty food, lethargy, generalized swelling, breast tenderness, abdominal bloating, swelling of the face or hands or feet, weight gain, headache, and change in bowel habits. Subjects were eliminated if their symptoms were present in the first half of the cycle or persisted for more than 2 days after onset of menses. Also excluded were pregnant women, psychiatric patients, and patients taking any drugs or medication, including oral contraceptives, for 4 weeks preceding the study.

Each participant completed the Menstrual Distress Questionnaire (MDQ) on days 7 and 25 of the menstrual cycle. The MDQ has been validated in three samples of women without PMS, and the normative values of both the premenstrual and the postmenstrual weeks have been reported (Moos, 1968). To evaluate symptom consistency, the MDQ was completed for three consecutive cycles (Chuong et al., 1980). Women whose scores on the MDQ were >80 on day 7 or <95 on day 25 were excluded from the PMS sample. Those with MDQ scores >80 on day 7 or >94 on day 25 were not accepted as control subjects.

EVALUATION OF PSYCHOLOGIC STATUS

The MMPI is a 550-item, self-report questionnaire containing items that describe feelings, attitudes, physical and emotional symptoms, and previous life experiences (Hathaway & McKinley, 1940). MMPI items have been grouped into scales by statistical means, and the patient's responses yield a profile of information about personality functioning and general mental health. The MMPI has become the most widely used and thoroughly researched of the objective personality assessment instruments currently available, and its application to patients with PMS is increasing (Lubin, Larsen, & Matarazzo, 1984; Hain et al., 1970; Gruba & Rohrbaugh, 1975; Muse et al., 1984; Stout & Steege, 1985; Steege, Stout, & Rupp, 1985; Hammond & Keye, Jr., 1985; Keye, Jr., Hammond, & Strong, 1986). Although the MMPI had its inception in 1937 and its norms are based on the responses of normal people from the late 1930s and early 1940s, data from a contemporary normal reference sample have recently been used to develop new norms for evaluating MMPI profiles (Colligan et al., 1983). Using these new norms has allowed us to make comparisons between our contemporary PMS sample and a contemporary sample of MMPI norms for women from 45 years ago.

Women in both the study and control groups completed the MMPI two times—on day 7 and day 25 of their menstrual cycle. MMPI profiles from the two groups were evaluated in several ways. First, the profiles from the women in our control group were compared with profiles from a census-matched sample of contemporary normal women whose MMPIs had been completed without regard for phase of the menstrual cycle (Colligan et al., 1983). This comparison ensured that MMPI response patterns from members of our small control group were comparable to the patterns of contemporary normal women in general. Separate comparisons were made for the follicular and luteal phases of the cycle. Also, the possibility that cyclical changes in psychologic status could occur among members of the control group was investigated by comparisons between the luteal and the follicular phases of the cycle. Second, MMPI profiles from our PMS patients were compared with those from the control group separately for the follicular and luteal phases of the cycle. Third, our PMS patients were compared with the census-matched sample of normal women (Colligan et al., 1983) during both the follicular and the luteal phases of their menstrual cycles. Finally, the changes in MMPI response patterns obtained during the follicular and luteal phases of the menstrual cycle were investigated in the PMS patients.

Because the statistical assumptions of (1) equal variances of scores between the PMS and control groups and (2) normal distributions (especially for evaluation of intracycle differences) could not be met for many of the MMPI scales under study, nonparametric tests based on median values—rather than means— were used for all scales (Snedecor & Cochran, 1967). Specifically, the signed-rank test was used for comparisons with the contemporary normal reference sample and for intracycle comparisons. The rank-sum test was used for comparisons between the PMS patients and the controls. Two-sided p values $\leq .05$ were reported as significant.

Table 11-1   Age, Marital Status, and Reproductive and Menstrual Histories of Patients with Premenstrual Syndrome (PMS) and of Control Subjects

	Control	PMS
Age (yr)		
Median	31.5	33.0
Range	19–42	22–48
Marital status (%)		
Single	20	15
Married	70	85
Divorced	10	0
Reproductive history (%)		
Nulliparous	45	40
Parous	55	60
Menstrual history (median)		
Menarche (yr)	12.4	12.7
Interval (days)	28.0	29.0
Length (days)	5.0	5.0
Dysmenorrhea (%)[a]		
None	25	10
Mild	60	15
Moderate	15	45
Severe	0	30

[a]$p < 0.001$.

RESULTS

There were no significant differences in age, marital status, reproductive history, or menstrual history between the PMS and the control groups (Table 11-1). However, more patients with PMS (75%) than controls (15%) reported moderate to severe dysmenorrhea.

Control Group: Comparison with Contemporary Normal Women

MMPI profiles from all members of the control group were well within normal limits during both follicular and luteal phases of the menstrual cycle. However, median t score values (Table 11-2) were significantly different from contemporary norms for women during the follicular phase on scales F, K, 1(Hs), 2(D), 6(Pa), 7(Pt), and 0(Si) and during the luteal phase on scales F, K, 1(Hs), 2(D), 6(Pa), 7(Pt), and 0(Si).

Both sets of profiles from our control subjects were completely within the expected range of values for contemporary Midwest women. However, members of our control group had described themselves as being more socially outgoing, having fewer physical complaints, and feeling less tension, anxiety, and worry than did the subjects participating in the 1983 MMPI normative study.

Control Group: Intracycle Changes

There were only minor changes in MMPI profiles from the follicular to the luteal phase of the menstrual cycle in the control group (Table 11-2). None of these median changes was of clinical or statistical (all p values $> .05$) significance, nor was any in the psychopathologic direction.

PMS Study Group: Comparisons with Control Group and Contemporary Normal Women—Follicular Phase

The median t score value for scale 6(Pa) in the PMS patients was significantly higher than the 1983 norm for women (Table 11-2). Median scores on scales F, 2(D), 6(Pa), and 7(Pt) were significantly higher in the PMS group than in our control group (Table 11-2).

Table 11-2   MMPI Median t Scores[a] by Day of Cycle and Median Intracycle Change in t Scores for Patients with PMS and Control Subjects

| | Day 7 (follicular) | | | Day 25 (luteal) | | | Day 7–day 25 | |
| | | | Control vs. PMS | | | Control vs. PMS | Intracycle changes | |
Scale	Control (median)	PMS (median)	(Rank-sum p value)	Control (median)	PMS (median)	(Rank-sum p value)	Control (median)	PMS (median)
L	51	46	>.20	46	46[b]	>.20	0	2
F	46[d]	51	.043	39[d]	57[d]	<.0001	0	−7[d]
K	57[d]	52	.12	59[d]	44[b]	<.0001	−1	9[d]
1(Hs)	45[d]	50	.056	46[b]	51	.0039	0	−2[b]
2(D)	44[d]	51	.013	41[d]	60[d]	<.0001	0	−9[d]
3(Hy)	53	51	>.20	50	60[d]	.0023	0	−7[d]
4(Pd)	54	53	>.20	51	61[d]	.0009	0	−6[d]
5(Mf)	52	45	>.20	47	44	>.20	2	2
6(Pa)	48[c]	56[b]	.0017	46[c]	61[d]	.0001	0	−6[d]
7(Pt)	46[c]	53	.016	47[b]	60[d]	.0008	−2	−6[d]
8(Sc)	46	51	>.20	48	52[b]	.025	−2	−7[d]
9(Ma)	50	54	>.20	48	55	.059	0	−2
0(Si)	40[d]	45	.10	38[b]	54	.0002	2	−5[d]

[a]All t scores are based on the contemporary adult norms (which have a median of 50).
[b]Signed-rank test of t score different from 50 (zero for day 7–day 25) is significant with $.02 < p \le .05$.
[c]Signed-rank test of t score different from 50 (zero for day 7–day 25) is significant with $.01 < p \le .02$.
[d]Signed-rank test of t score different from 50 (zero for day 7–day 25) is significant with $p \le .01$.

Clinically, these differences indicated significant feelings of interpersonal oversensitivity and the increased likelihood of having one's feelings hurt by others. Significant feelings of depression, tension, and anxiety were also reported, all in comparison with the 1983 norms and with our control group. Indeed, for 5 PMS patients (25%), further evaluation of their mental health was indicated from the profile.

PMS Study Group: Intracycle Changes

Numerous significant MMPI changes from the follicular to the luteal phase were found among members of the PMS group (Table 11-2). Less effective psychologic functioning and increased psychologic stress (Figure 11-1) were observed when the luteal-phase values were compared with the follicular-phase results.

Median scores on all clinical scales except 5(Mf) and 9(Ma) increased significantly (Table 11-2). Among the validity scales, F increased significantly and K decreased significantly. This change in validity-scale configuration suggested a lowering of the psychologic defenses or ego strength available to the individual and an accompanying tendency to report more symptoms.

PMS Study Group: Comparisons with Control Group and Normal Contemporary Women—Luteal Phase

In the PMS patients, median t score values were significantly different from the 1983 MMPI norms for women in scales L, F, K, 2(D), 3(Hy), 4(Pd), 6(Pa), 7(Pt), and 8(Sc) (Table 11-2). In comparison with scores attained by members of the control sample, median t score values for the PMS group were significantly different for scales F, K, 1(Hs), 2(D), 3(Hy), 4(Pd), 6(Pa), 7(Pt), 8(Sc), and 0(Si) (Table 11-2).

For some patients, these profiles indicated an exacerbation of the significant symptoms reported during the follicular phase. For others, a set of symptoms completely foreign to the individual during the follicular phase appeared during the luteal phase. In general, the mean profile (Figure 11-1) for PMS patients during the luteal phase was characterized by significant feelings of overall stress, tension, depression, anxiety, nervousness, oversensitivity, and social discomfort. For 10 of the patients, these symptoms were severe enough to indicate further evaluation of mental health status.

DISCUSSION

In addition to the routine physical examination and laboratory studies, it is equally important to assess the severity and cyclical variation, if any, of the psychologic symptoms that accompany the physiologic changes during the men-

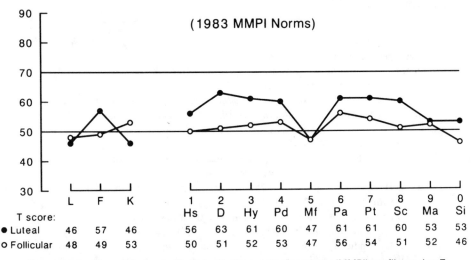

Figure 11-1 Mean Minnesota Multiphasic Personality Inventory (MMPI) profile on day 7 (follicular phase) and day 25 (luteal phase) of the menstrual cycle for 20 women with premenstrual syndrome.

strual cycle. The relationship between PMS changes and underlying psychologic problems or psychiatric disorders has long been reported (Endo et al., 1978; Halbreich, Endicott, & Nee, 1983; Halbreich & Endicott, 1985), and the difficulties associated with carrying out meaningful PMS research are well documented (Gannon, 1981; Rubinow & Roy-Byrne, 1984). However, the data from our study are consistent with those recently offered from a pilot project (Trunnell, Rote, & Keye, Jr., 1985). These data suggest that although the MMPI is useful in evaluating patients with PMS, it is essential that clinicians be aware of the point in the menstrual cycle at which the MMPI is completed by the patient.

Our MMPI data, although from a small sample, are buttressed by comparisons with a control group and a large sample of contemporary normal women, and they also suggest the existence of two PMS subgroups. The first has cyclical variations—from completely normal MMPI values during the follicular phase to significantly dysfunctional levels during the luteal phase. The second subgroup has psychologic stress and dysfunction throughout the cycle that are significantly greater than those in women without PMS, and the symptoms are exacerbated during the luteal phase. From 25 to 50% of our PMS patients had MMPI profiles indicating a need for further evaluation of mental health, perhaps through psychiatric interview (Harrison, Rabkin, & Endicott, 1985). Different treatment approaches are likely to be needed for these two subgroups, especially if a concomitant psychiatric problem is identified.

REFERENCES

Chuong, C. J., Coulam, C. B., Kao, P. C., Bergstralh, E. J., & Go, V. L. W. (1980). Neuropeptide levels in premenstrual syndrome. *Fertility and Sterility, 44,* 760–765.

Colligan, R. C., Osborne, D., Swenson, W. M., & Offord, K. P. (1983). *The MMPI: A contemporary normative study.* New York: Praeger.

Endo, M., Daiguji, M., Asano, Y., et al. (1978). Periodic psychosis recurring in association with menstrual cycle. *Journal of Clinical Psychiatry, 39,* 456–466.

Frank, R. T. (1931). The hormonal causes of premenstrual tension. *Archives of Neurological Psychiatry, 26,* 1053–1057.

Gannon, L. (1981). Evidence for a psychological etiology of menstrual disorders: A critical review. *Psychology Report, 48,* 287–294.

Gruba, G. H., & Rohrbaugh, M. (1975). MMPI correlates of menstrual distress. *Psychosomatic Medicine, 37,* 265–273.

Hain, J. D., Linton, P. H., Eber, H. W., et al. (1970). Menstrual irregularity, symptoms and personality. *Journal of Psychosomatic Research, 14,* 81–87.

Halbreich, U., Endicott, J., & Nee, J. (1983). Premenstrual depressive changes: Value of differentiation. *Archives of General Psychiatry, 40,* 535–542.

Halbreich, U., & Endicott, J. (1985). Relationship of dysphoric premenstrual changes to depressive disorders. *Acta Psychiatrica Scandinavica, 71,* 331–338.

Hammond, D. C., & Keye, Jr., W. R. (1985). Premenstrual syndrome (letter to the editor). *New England Journal of Medicine, 312,* 920.

Harrison, W. M., Rabkin, J. G., & Endicott, J. (1985). Psychiatric evaluation of premenstrual changes. *Psychosomatics, 26,* 789–799.

Hathaway, S. R., & McKinley, J. C. (1940). A multiphasic personality schedule (Minnesota). I. Construction of the schedule. *Journal of Psychology, 10,* 249–254.

Keye, Jr., W. R., Hammond, D. C., & Strong, T. (1986). Medical and psychological characteristics of women presenting with premenstrual symptoms. *Obstetrics and Gynecology, 68,* 634–637.

Lubin, B., Larsen, R. M., & Matarazzo, J. D. (1984). Patterns of psychological test usage in the United States: 1935–1982. *American Psychology, 39,* 451–454.

Moos, R. H. (1968). The development of a menstrual distress questionnaire. *Psychosomatic Medicine, 30,* 853–867.

Muse, K. N., Cetel, N. S., Futterman, L. A., et al. (1984). The premenstrual syndrome: Effects of "medical ovariectomy." *New England Journal of Medicine, 311,* 1345–1349.

Rubinow, D. R., & Roy-Byrne, P. (1984). Premenstrual syndromes: Overview from a methodologic perspective. *American Journal of Psychiatry, 141,* 163–172.

Snedecor, G. W., & Cochran, W. G. (1967). *Statistical methods* (6th ed.) (pp. 100–102). Ames, IA: Iowa State University Press.

Steege, J. F., Stout, A. L., & Rupp, S. L. (1985). Relationships among premenstrual symptoms and menstrual cycle characteristics. *Obstetrics and Gynecology, 65,* 398–402.

Stout, A. L., & Steege, J. F. (1985). Psychological assessment of women seeking treatment for premenstrual syndrome. *Journal of Psychosomatic Research, 29,* 621–629.

Trunnell, E., Rote, N., & Keye, W. R. (1985). Influence of menstrual cycle phase on psychometric testing in women with premenstrual syndrome (PMS). Presented at 32nd annual meeting of the Society for Gynecologic Investigation, Phoenix, Arizona, March 20–23, 1985. *Scientific Program and Abstracts,* p. 342P.

Chapter 12

A Survey of Multidimensional and Interdisciplinary Approaches to Premenstrual Syndrome

Mary Ellen Robertson

INTRODUCTION

Premenstrual syndrome (PMS) is the cyclic occurrence of a physical and behavioral cluster of signs and symptoms, and its prevalence is being recognized in clinical settings (Hargrove & Abraham, 1982, 1983; Woods, Most, & Dery, 1982a). Over 150 symptoms have been associated with premenstrual syndrome. A variety of biochemical and psychosocial elements have been explored in the literature to identify the etiology and pathophysiology of PMS. Strategies that have been implemented to combat the signs and symptoms of PMS include support groups, nutrition therapy, exercise therapy, stress management, and an array of pharmacotherapeutic agents. Because of the elusive etiology, the complexity of the symptomatology, and the variety of treatment modalities being employed, a challenge exists to create services for PMS that are individualistic and multidimensional. A survey was conducted of a sample of 40 PMS centers that offer services to women who suffer from PMS, to identify the interdisciplinary professionals who provide service, the screening procedures used at the centers, the treatment modalities being employed, and the professionals to which these centers refer women suffering from PMS.

Definition of PMS

The term premenstrual tension was coined by Frank in 1931, who described 15 patients with nervous tension, edema, and weight gain, of whom 11 improved markedly after menses. Since then, there has been a growing awareness of the incidence of premenstrual tension syndrome. Definition of PMS is broad and vague, usually encompassing a cluster of signs and symptoms, which reoccur cyclically in a premenstrual interval (London, Sundaram, Murphy, & Goldstein, 1983; Reid & Yen, 1981). This difficulty in defining PMS is a result of the variety of combinations of more than 150 symptoms described in relation to PMS.

Etiology

In spite of attempts to identify PMS's pathophysiology, its etiology remains uncompleted. The role of ovarian steroids has been examined, suggesting a lowered progesterone level in relation to a higher estrogen level (Backstrom & Carstensen, 1974; Dalton, 1964, 1984; Mundy, 1977, 1981; Norris, 1983). In addition, prolactin levels were investigated in relation to PMS (Labrum, 1979, 1983; Steiner, 1984). Studies on the use of bromocriptine to lower prolactin levels showed conflicting results (Elsner, 1980; Ylostalo, Kauppila, & Puolakka, 1982; Steiner, 1984). Andersch and Hahn (1982), in a double-blind, placebo-controlled study, found no significant difference with bromocriptine, but had some differences reported in breast symptoms. Chihal (1985) reported that the side effects of the bromocriptine were in some cases worse than the PMS symptoms.

Fluctuating serotonin levels, resulting from estrogen negative feedback, have also been described in the literature in relation to PMS (Taylor, Mathew, & Ho, 1982). Reid and Yen (1981; Reid, 1983) suggest a beta-endorphin and alpha-melanocyte withdrawal, which in turn causes neuroendocrine changes resulting in behavioral manifestations.

Nutritional deficiencies such as vitamin B and vitamin A have also been theorized in the etiology of PMS (Abraham & Hargrove, 1980; Abraham & Lubran, 1981; Abraham, Schwartz, & Lubran, 1984; Argonz & Abinzano, 1950; Biskind, Biskind, & Biskind, 1944; Goei & Abraham, 1983; Goei, Ralston, & Abraham, 1982).

In addition, there exist conflicting results in the relationship of psychological or social disorder in association with PMS (Berry & McGuire, 1972; Coppen & Kessel, 1963; Henricksen, 1962). Woods (1985) found a positive relationship between current incidence of perimenstrual symptoms and negative attitudes about menstruation.

Diagnostic Techniques

Due to the cluster of emotional, behavioral, and physical symptoms involved in PMS, diagnostic techniques are multidimensional. Standardized rating scales are used to identify symptoms and assess severity. Moos (1968) developed a menstrual distress questionnaire, a retrospective tool, to assess changes in the menstrual cycle. This questionnaire was modified by Abraham (1980) to include a clustering of symptoms: PMT-A (nervous tension, mood swings, irritability, and anxiety); PMT-H (sensation of weight gain, swelling of extremities, breast tenderness, and abdominal bloating); PMT-C (headache, craving for sweets, increased appetite, heart pounding, fatigue, and dizziness); and PMT-D (depression, forgetfulness, easy crying, confusion, insomnia). Abraham bases his treatment on the category that applies to the client's symptomatology. Prospective rating scales in the form of the client's daily recording of symptoms, such as a menstrual symptom diary, have also been described in the assessment of the PMS client (Youngs, 1986). Halbreich, Endicott, and Schacht (1982) studied 48 women and found a significant difference in the recordings of the severity of reported symptoms in the retrospective recordings and the daily menstrual cycle diary. Symptoms were less severe in the daily reports.

Recommendations for the assessment and management of PMS have also been included in the literature. Chihal (1985) outlines a procedure for clinical management of the PMS client, which includes a complete history, physical examination, suicide risk evaluation, menstrual cycle symptom diary, psychological testing (Zung's anxiety and depression scales are suggested), diet, and exercise assessment. Lauersen and Stukane (1983) include lab screening encompassing CBC, SMA-12, FSH/LH ratio, serum estradiol, serum progesterone, serum prolactin, and T and T in the PMS assessment. Youngs (1986) includes psychometric assessment using the Hopkin's Symptom Checklist. Keye (1985) suggests psychologic testing to assist in differential diagnosis of PMS.

Impact on the family has also been reported in the literature (Brown & Zimmer, 1986; Dalton, 1964). Brown and Zimmer (1986) found family disruption in a study of 83 women and 32 men with PMS in their family. A more indepth and careful documentation of the impact of PMS on the family was called for by these two researchers. Based on these findings, family assessment could also be included in the screening of the PMS client.

Treatment

The following is a sampling of the treatment modalities, which have been described in the literature, to emphasize that a variety of modalities are being explored. This is not a critical review of research designs to test these modalities. This researcher recognizes the limitations of uncontrolled studies and refers to critical review of these research studies (Coyne, Woods, & Mitchell,

1986; Duncan & Amorosino, 1984; Rowe, 1985; Rubinow & Roy-Byrne, 1984; Steiner, Haskett, & Carroll, 1980).

Because of the elusive etiology of PMS, treatment modalities have varied in scope and research. As previously discussed, bromocriptine has been studied in relation to dopamine and prolactin levels for the treatment of PMS (Andersch & Hahn, 1982). Progesterone therapy has been suggested in the literature, and trials using double-blind, placebo-controlled designs have shown no significant difference in PMS symptoms (Sampson, 1979), yet Dalton (1983, 1984) successfully treated women using this modality. Danazol, a synthetic androgen, has been identified as effective because of the inhibition of the pituitary-ovarian axis, but its side effects have also been criticized in the literature (Chihal, 1985).

Antiprostaglandin therapy has been suggested as a second-line choice and found effective in a study by Wood and Jakubowicz (1980) using mefenamic acid. Spirolactone as studied by Hendler (1980) is used as an antagonist for aldosterone and has improved PMS symptoms in 6 out of 7 clients in the trial. Antagonists of gonadotropin-releasing hormone, studied by Muse, Cetel, Futterman, and Yen (1984), showed marked improvement in 8 PMS clients. Other pharmacotherapeutic agents suggested include antidepressants and antianxiety medication. Nutrition and vitamin/mineral supplementation is widely discussed in the literature (Abraham & Hargrove, 1980; Abraham, 1980a, 1980b; Abraham, Schwartz, & Lubran, 1984; Abraham & Lubran, 1981; Block, 1960; Goei & Abraham, 1983; Goei, Ralston, & Abraham, 1982; Shangold, 1982). Exercise therapy has also been prescribed for PMS clients as a stress reduction technique and aerobic conditioning (Timonen & Procope, 1971).

Purpose of the Study

Because of the unknown etiology of PMS and the conflicting results of treatment modalities in the literature, the question could be asked what is currently being done to assist women who have PMS and what professionals are providing that service? This survey attempts to describe current practices in a sample of PMS centers in the United States, but does not attempt to interpret efficacy of treatment modalities. Four areas of investigation are addressed in this survey:

1 What types of professionals intervene with the PMS clients at the PMS centers?

2 What screening procedures are employed for assessment of the PMS client?

3 What types of professionals are PMS clients referred to for the treatment of their PMS?

4 What treatment modalities are employed for the management of PMS clients at the PMS centers?

This survey identifies the types of professional personnel at a sample of PMS centers that are providing services for PMS clients and the multidimensional approaches to screening and treatment.

METHODOLOGY

A sample of 40 PMS centers were randomly selected to participate in the study from a list of United States centers that provide assessment and treatment of PMS clients. Participation in the survey was voluntary, and respondents were assured anonymity. Of the 40 surveys sent to centers, 5 were returned because of no forwarding address. Of the 35 remaining centers, 26 responded to the survey, resulting in a response rate of 74%.

Data analysis consisted of frequency determination of personnel, referrals, screening procedures, and treatment modalities reported by the centers.

RESULTS

What Types of Professionals Intervene with PMS Clients at PMS Centers?

The mean number of PMS center personnel was 3.42, with physicians accounting for the greatest number (76.9%) (Table 12-1a). The physician specialty most frequently reported was obstetrician-gynecologist (53.8%) (Table 12-1b). General practitioners (15.4%), psychiatrists (11.5%), endocrinologists (7.7%), and naturopathic physicians (7.7%) were also reported.

Eleven categories of professional personnel were identified in the survey (Tables 12-1a & 12-1c). These included nurse practitioners (34.6%), social workers (26.9%), registered nurses (26.9%), psychologists (19.2%), support group leaders (11.5%), family counselors (7.7%), and chiropractors (7.7%). Support group leaders varied among psychotherapists, nurses, educators, counselors, and social service personnel.

What Types of Professionals Are PMS Clients Referred to for the Treatment of Their PMS?

The centers reported a mean total of 3.73 types of personnel to whom they refer PMS clients. Nine categories of personnel were identified for referral, which included nutritionists (53.8%), support groups (46.2%), psychologists (42.3%), exercise programs (38.5%), marriage counselors (38.5%), family therapists (26.9%), nurse practitioners (19.2%), and chiropractors (19.2%) (Tables 12-2a & 12-2b). The physician category for referrals included obstetrician-gynecologists (65.3%), psychiatrists (46.1%), endocrinologists (38.5%), general practitioners (34.6%), internists (3.8%), and PMS specialists

Table 12-1a   Types of Personnel at PMS Centers

Personnel	No.	%
Physician	20	76.9
Nutritionist	11	42.3
Nurse practitioner	9	34.6
Social worker	7	26.9
Registered nurse	7	26.9
Psychologist	5	19.2

n = 26.

Table 12-1b   Number of Physician Specialties at PMS Centers

Physicians	No.	%
OB-GYN	14	53.8
General practitioner	4	15.4
Psychiatrist	3	11.5
Endocrinologist	2	7.7
Other	2	7.7

n = 26.

Table 12-1c   Types of Personnel at PMS Centers

Personnel	No.	%
Support group leader	3	11.5
Exercise therapist	3	11.5
LPN	3	11.5
Family counselor	2	7.7
Chiropractor	2	7.7

n = 26.

(3.8%) (Table 12-2c). Total personnel and total referral figures for the PMS centers are listed in Table 12-2d.

What Screening Procedures Are Employed for Assessment of the PMS Client?

The mean total of screening modalities for PMS clients at these centers was 7.26. Self-rating symptom charting (96.2%), diet history (92.3%), exercise history (84.6%), and medical history (80.8%) were the most frequent screening tools reported, followed by physical exam (65.4%) and lab screening (61.5%) (Table 12-3a). Lab screening included thyroid function testing (57.7%), SMAC (42.3%), urinalysis (38.4%), glucose (30.7%), FSH/LH ratio (36.9%), prolactin (26.9%), and progesterone (23.0%) (Table 12-3b). Psychosocial screening included suicide risk (42.3%), marital assessment (38.5%), psychologic testing (23.0%), and personality testing (19.1%) (Table 12-3c). The centers reported the use of Beck's Depression Inventory, Hamilton Anxiety and Depression Scales, and Holmes Rahe Life Stress Assessment and Alcohol Use Inventory. Total screening modality figures are noted in Table 12-3d.

Table 12-2a Type of Referrals for PMS Clients

Referral	No.	%
Nutritionist	14	53.8
Support groups	12	46.2
Psychologist	11	42.3
Exercise program	10	38.5
Marriage counselor	10	38.5

$n = 26$.

Table 12-2b Type of Referrals for PMS Clients

Family therapist	7	26.9
Nurse practitioner	5	19.2
Chiropractor	5	19.2

$n = 26$.

Table 12-2c Types of Physicians for PMS Referrals

Physicians	No. of referring centers	%
OB-GYN	17	65.3
General practitioner	9	34.6
Endocrinologist	10	38.5
Psychiatrist	13	46.1
Other	2	7.7

$n = 26$.

Table 12-2d Total Personnel and Total Referrals

Mean	SD	Variance
Total Personnel at PMS Centers		
3.42	1.77	3.13
Total Referrals Made at PMS Centers		
3.73	2.58	6.68

Table 12-3a   Screening Procedures at PMS Centers

Screening	No.	%
Client symptom charting	25	96.2
Diet history	24	92.3
Exercise history	22	84.6
Medical history	21	80.8
Physical exam	17	65.4
Lab screening	16	61.5

$n = 26.$

Table 12-3b   Lab Screening at PMS Centers

Lab	No.	%
Thyroid	15	57.7
SMAC	11	42.3
Urinalysis	10	38.4
Glucose	9	30.7
FSH/LH	7	26.9
Prolactin	7	26.9
Progesterone	6	23.0

Table 12-3c   Screening Procedures at PMS Centers

Screening	No.	%
Suicide risk	11	42.3
Marital assessment	10	38.5
Basal body temperature (BBT)	8	30.8
Psychological testing	6	23.0
Personality testing	5	19.1

$n = 26.$

Table 12-3d   Total Screening Modalities

Mean	SD	Variance
7.26	2.53	6.44

What Treatment Modalities Are Employed for the Management of PMS Clients at the PMS Centers?

The mean total treatment modalities reported by the centers for PMS clients was 3.88. Vitamin/mineral supplementation and diet therapy was the primary treatment, both at 92.3% (Table 12-4a). Combination of vitamins and minerals varied (Table 12-4b). Exercise therapy was reported in 76.9% of the PMS centers.

Pharmacotherapeutic agents that the centers identified in their treatment programs included progesterone (80.7%), diuretics (57.6%), antidepressants (38.4%), analgesics (38.4%), and antiprostaglandins (38.4%) (Table 12-4c). Acupuncture/acupressor was included in 7.7% of the centers and biofeedback at 19.2%.

Psychosocial modalities included psychologic services (61.5%), support groups (53.8%), marriage counseling (34.6%), and child counseling (19.2%) (Table 12-4d). Total treatment modality figures are listed in Table 12-4e.

DISCUSSION

The results of the survey confirm the use of interdisciplinary and multidimensional approaches to PMS. Eleven categories of personnel at the PMS centers point out the variety of professionals working with PMS clients, in addition to the referral to nine other categories of personnel. Although physicians were reported most often, many professional disciplines were represented. The high percentage of referral to nutritionists supports the etiologic theory regarding dietary deficiencies and the use of diet therapy in the treatment of PMS.

With the number of professionals encountered by the PMS client during treatment, further investigation is needed to clarify coordination of services.

Table 12-4a   Treatment Modalities Used at PMS Centers

Treatments	No.	%
Vitamin/mineral	24	92.3
Diet therapy	24	92.3
Exercise therapy	20	76.9
Psychological services	16	61.5
Support groups	14	53.8

Table 12-4b   Vitamins/Minerals

	No.	%
Optivite	8	30.8
Vitamin A	13	50.0
Vitamin B complex	17	65.4
Vitamin C	11	42.3
Vitamin D	12	46.3
Vitamin E	14	53.8
Magnesium	13	50.0
Calcium	14	53.8

Table 12-4c   Treatment Modalities Used at PMS Centers

RX	No.	%
Progesterone	21	80.7
Diuretics	15	57.6
Antidepressants	10	38.4
Analgesics	10	38.4
Antiprostaglandins	10	38.4

$n = 26.$

Table 12-4d   Treatment Modalities Used at PMS Centers

Treatment	No.	%
Marriage counseling	9	34.6
Evening primrose oil	7	26.9
Biofeedback	5	19.2
Child counseling	5	19.2
Acupuncture/acupressor	2	7.7

$n = 26.$

Table 12-4e   Total Treatment Modalities

Mean	SD	Variance
3.88	2.08	4.34

One question to be asked is who should coordinate services for the client with PMS, and is a client advocate available to increase communication among professionals or does care get fragmented?

Nine categories of professionals who could receive referrals of PMS clients from the centers reflect the variety of treatment recommendations and etiologic theories that are found in clinical and research literature, in addition to the complexity of symptoms that may be identified in the PMS client. Further investigation of criteria used to determine the need for referral and to what type of professional for what type of service is needed. In addition, another question to ask is, what is the cost these services to the PMS client?

Self-reporting of menstrual symptoms was the most frequent screening tool used by the centers, followed by diet history, exercise history, and medical history. Lab screening was used in over half of the centers; however, there was little consistency in the types of lab tests being performed, except that 57.7% of the 61.5% of centers performing lab screening performed a thyroid function test. Further investigation is needed for criteria for types of lab screening.

Of the treatment modalities used, there was a high percentage of centers using diet therapy with vitamin supplementation (92.3%). Progesterone was the leading pharmacotherapeutic agent identified (80.7%), despite conflicting results on efficacy reported in the literature.

Of the psychosocial modalities used, less than half the centers included psychological screening; however, 61.5% of the centers identified some type of psychologic service that could be provided. Screening for effect on the family was not highly identified, with only 38.5% of the centers identifying some type of marital assessment and only 34.6% of the centers identifying marriage counseling. Child intervention for children of PMS clients was only identified in 19.2% of the centers.

This survey identified the multidimensional and interdisciplinary approaches to PMS assessment and treatment using a sample of PMS centers in the United States. The variety of personnel, screening, and treatment modalities reflects those found in clinical and research literature. As PMS research evolves, there may be even more diversity as new theories of etiology and treatment are researched. Because of this diversity, it is important that the PMS client seeking assistance is well informed on the screening, treatment, and referral plan, and the centers should make efforts to coordinate these modalities.

A question not asked in the survey, which should be addressed, is how many of the centers are doing research on PMS to contribute to the existing body of knowledge about PMS? Another research question to consider is, what criteria are used to determine types of personnel, screening, treatment modalities, and referrals to be used in assessment and treatment of the PMS client?

REFERENCES

Abraham, G. E. (1980a) Premenstrual tension. In M. Leventhal (Ed.), *Current problems in obstetrics and gynecology* (pp. 1–48). Chicago: Year Book Medical Publishers.

Abraham, G. E. (1980b). The premenstrual tension syndrome. *Obstetric Gynecologic Nursing, 3*(1).

Abraham, G. E., & Hargrove, J. T. (1980). Effects of vitamin B_6 on premenstrual symptomatology in women with premenstrual tension syndrome: A double blind crossover study. *Infertility, 2,* 315.

Abraham, G. E., & Lubran, M. M. (1981). Serum and red cell magnesium levels in patients with premenstrual tension. *American Journal of Clinical Nutrition, 34,* 2364.

Abraham, G. E., Schwartz, U. D., & Lubran, M. M. (1984). Effect of B_6 on plasma and red blood cell magnesium levels in premenopausal women. *Annals of Clinical and Laboratory Science, 11,* 333–336.

Andersch, B., & Hahn, L. (1982). Bromocriptine and premenstrual tension, a clinical and hormonal study. *Pharmatherapeutica, 3,* 107.

Argonz, J., & Abinzano, C. (1950). Premenstrual tension treated with vitamin A. *Journal of Clinical Endocrinal Metabolism, 10,* 572.

Backstrom, T., & Carstensen, H. (1974). Estrogen and progesterone in plasma in relation to premenstrual tension. *Journal of Steroid Biochemistry, 5,* 257.

Berry, C., & McGuire, F. L. (1972). Menstrual distress and acceptance of sexual role. *American Journal of Obstetrics and Gynecology, 114,* 83.

Biskind, M. S., Biskind, G. R., & Biskind, L. H. (1944). Nutritional deficiency in the etiology of menorrhagia, metrorrhagia, cystic mastitis and premenstrual tension. *Surgical Gynecology and Obstetrics, 78,* 49.

Block, E. (1960). The use of vitamin A in premenstrual tension. *Acta Obstetrica et Gynecologica Scandinavica, 39*(16), 585.

Brown, M. A., & Zimmer, P. A. (1986). Personal and family impact of premenstrual symptoms. *Journal of Obstetric, Gynecologic, and Neonatal Nursing, 15*(1), 31–38.

Chihal, H. J. (1985). *Premenstrual syndrome: A clinic manual.* Durant, OK: Creative Informatics, Inc.

Coppen, A., & Kessel, N. (1963). Menstruation and personality. *British Journal of Psychiatry, 109,* 711.

Coyne, C. M., Woods, N. F., & Mitchell, E. S. (1985). Premenstrual tension syndrome. *Journal of Obstetric, Gynecologic, and Neonatal Nursing, 14*(6), 446–453.

Dalton, K. (1964). *The premenstrual syndrome.* Springfield, IL: Charles C Thomas.

Dalton, K. (1983). *Once a month.* Clemont, CA: Hunter House.

Dalton, K. (1984). *The premenstrual syndrome and progesterone therapy* (2nd ed.). Chicago, IL: Yearbook Medical Publishers, Inc.

Duncan, F. J., & Amorosino, C. S. (1984). Premenstrual syndrome. *The New England Journal of Medicine, 311,* 1371–1373.

Elsner, C. (1980). Bromocryptines in the treatment of premenstrual tension syndrome. *Obstetrics and Gynecology, 56,* 723.

Frank, R. T. (1931). The hormonal causes of premenstrual tension. *Archives of Neurologic Psychiatry, 26,* 1053.

Goei, G. S., & Abraham, G. E. (1983). Effect of nutritional supplements, optivite, on symptoms of premenstrual tension. *Journal of Reproductive Medicine, 28,* 527–531.

Goei, G. S., Ralston, J. L., & Abraham, G. E. (1982). Dietary patterns of patients with premenstrual tension. *Journal of Applied Nutrition, 34,* 4.

Halbreich, U., Endicott, J., & Schacht, S. (1982). Premenstrual assessment form: A new procedure to reflect the diversity of premenstrual changes. *Acta Psychiatrica Scandinavica, 65,* 46.

Hargrove, J. T., & Abraham, G. E. (1982). The incidence of premenstrual tension in a gynecological clinic. *Journal of Reproductive Medicine, 28,* 721.

Hargrove, J. T., & Abraham, G. E. (1983). The ubiquitousness of premenstrual tension in gynecologic practice. *Journal of Reproductive Medicine,* 435–437.

Hendler, N. H. (1980). Clinical drug trial spironolactone for premenstrual syndrome. *The Female Patient, 5,* 17.

Henriksen, E. (1962). The melancholies of menstruation or premenstrual tension. *Clinical OB-GYN, 5,* 252.

Keye, W. R. (1985). Psychological testing can clarify PMS. *OB-GYN News, 1*(14), 8.

Labrum, A. H. (1979). Prolactin and premenstrual syndrome. *The Female Patient, 4,* 76.

Labrum, A. H. (1983). Hypothalamic pireal and pituitary factors in PMS. *Journal of Reproductive Medicine, 28,* 438–445.

Lauersen, N. H. (1985, March). Recognition and treatment of premenstrual syndrome. *Nurse Practitioner,* pp. 11–22.

Lauersen, N. H., & Stukane, E. (1983). *Premenstrual syndrome and you.* New York: NY: Simon & Schuster, Inc.

London, R. S., Sundaram, G. S., Murphy, L., & Goldman, P. J. (1983). Evaluation and treatment of breast symptoms in patients with premenstrual syndrome. *Journal of Reproductive Medicine, 28,* 503–508.

Moos, R. H. (1968). The development of a menstrual distress questionnaire. *Psychosomatic Medicine, 30,* 853.

Mundy, M. (1977). Progesterone and aldosterone levels in premenstrual tension syndrome. *Journal of Endocrinology, 73,* 21.

Mundy, M. R., Brush, M. G., & Taylor, R. W. (1981). Correlations between progesterone, estradiol and aldosterone levels in premenstrual syndrome. *Clinical Endocrinology, 14,* 1.

Muse, K., Cetel, N. S., Futterman, L. A., & Yen, S. S. C. (1984). The premenstrual syndrome effects of medical ovariectomy. *New England Journal of Medicine, 311,* 1345.

Norris, R. V. (1983). Progesterone for premenstrual tension. *Journal of Reproductive Medicine, 28,* 509–524.

PMS News and Views (1986, Fall). Physician survey: Which treatment for PMS. *Chattem Bulletin for Physicians and Other Health Professionals,* pp. 1–5.

Rees, L. (1953). The premenstrual tension syndrome and its treatment. *British Medical Journal, 1,* 1014.

Reid, R. L. (1983). Endogenous opioid activity and premenstrual syndrome. *Lancet, ii,* 786.

Reid, R., & Yen, S. S. C. (1981). Premenstrual syndrome. *American Journal of Obstetrics and Gynecology, 139,* 85.

Rowe, T. C. (1985). Premenstrual syndrome: Theories and treatment. *Clinical GYN Briefs,* 1–4.

Rubinow, D. R., & Roy-Byrne, P. (1984). Premenstrual syndrome: Overview from a methodologic perspective. *American Journal of Psychiatry, 141,* 163.

Sampson, G. A. (1979). Premenstrual syndrome: A double-blind controlled trial and progesterone and placebo. *British Journal of Psychiatry, 135,* 209–215.

Shangold, M. M. (1982). PMS is real, but what can you do about it? *Contemporary OB/GYN, 19,* 251.

Steiner, M. (1984). Plasma prolactin and severe premenstrual tension. *Psychoneuroendocrinology, 9,* 29.

Steiner, M., Haskett, F. R., & Carroll, B. J. (1980). Premenstrual tension syndrome: The development of research diagnostic criteria and new rating scales. *Acta Psychiatrica Scandinavica, 62,* 177–190.

Taylor, D., Mathew, R. T., & Ho, B. T. (1982). Serotonin levels and platelet uptake during premenstrual tension. *Advanced Biochemical Psychopharmacology, 34,* 328.

Timonen, S., & Procope, B. (1971). Premenstrual syndrome and physical exercise. *Acta Obstetrica et Gynecologica Scandinavica, 50,* 331.

Wood, C., & Jakubowicz, P. (1980). The treatment of premenstrual tension with mefenamic acid. *British Journal of Obstetrics and Gynaecology, 627,* 87.

Woods, N. F. (1985). Relationship of socialization and stress to premenstrual symptoms, disability, and menstrual attitudes. *Nursing Research, 34,* 145–149.

Woods, N., Most, A., & Dery, G. (1982). Prevalence of perimenstrual symptoms. *American Journal of Public Health, 72,* 1257–1264.

Ylostalo, P., Kauppila, A., & Puolakka, J. (1982). Bromocriptine and norethisterone in the treatment of premenstrual syndrome. *Obstetrics and Gynecology, 59,* 292.

Youngs, D. D. (1986). Assessing premenstrual syndrome in a private practice setting. *Postgraduate Obstetrics and Gynecology, 6,* 1–6.

Chapter 13

Premenstrual Syndrome: A Bio-Psycho-Social Approach to Treatment

Peg Miota, Mary Yahle, and Carole Bartz

INTRODUCTION

Premenstrual syndrome (PMS) has been described as the disease of the '80s, "an illness from which more than three-quarters of women suffer" (Lever & Brush, 1981, p. 1). Little attention has been given to the differences between normal premenstrual changes, premenstrual symptoms, and the exacerbation of symptoms present at other times of the month. Professionals who treat PMS without such differentiation run several risks, including that of defining the normal menstrual cycle as a disease. Women who experience incapacitating premenstrual symptoms could have other problems that are exacerbated premenstrually.

Pregnancy and childbirth were treated as a disease in the late 1800s. In the United States it was not until 1950 that women began to recognize the need to regain control of the normal physiologic process of pregnancy and birth, and to insist on rights related to their minds and bodies. They demanded to be awake during childbirth, have their partner present, and assume a comfortable, unrestrained position during birthing. Women organized and attended childbirth classes taught by other women. They learned to understand what was happening to them physiologically, to care for themselves during pregnancy, and to cooperate with their bodies during childbirth. Currently, women are redefining menopause as a normal physiologic process rather than an illness. They are learning that most menopausal changes are normal and can be managed with good self-care.

The PMS Treatment Program at Milwaukee Psychiatric Hospital was established to provide women with the opportunity to manage and benefit from their natural menstrual experience. They do so by identifying their individual cyclic symptoms, assessing contributing physiologic, interpersonal, and sociocultural aspects, and making indicated life changes. This chapter describes the PMS Treatment Program at Milwaukee Psychiatric Hospital. This program was established to provide women with the opportunity to identify their individual cyclic symptoms, learn to reduce the severity of symptoms, develop an appreciation of the positive aspects of cyclical change, and use these new awarenesses to make necessary life changes.

THE ADAPTIVE FUNCTION OF PREMENSTRUAL SYMPTOMS

Every month from menarche to menopause, a woman's body prepares for pregnancy. Women experience multiple normal, measurable physical changes as part of that monthly preparation. Changes in behavior and feelings accompany and are related to the preparation for pregnancy. Asso (1983) suggests that specific changes in mood and behavior at the time of potential fertilization may enhance the complicated process of conception.

The sociocultural context within which a woman defines her reproductivity is superimposed on these physical, emotional, and behavioral changes. Women are choosing to have fewer children and an increasing number of women are opting for a child-free lifestyle. Women are therefore experiencing more periods during their life cycles. Women are learning new uses for monthly changes in feelings and behavior, which can now serve to enhance the monthly rebirth of the women themselves.

The PMS Treatment Program first considered the complications women experience trying to balance their biological processes with the sociocultural demands of contemporary society. In developing our treatment philosophy, we used our expertise as women and our clinical expertise.

Historically, women have sought help from professionals for physical symptoms often related to the reproductive system. Moreover, physical symptoms can be manifestations of intense emotional needs. In a patriarchal society, physical symptoms are more acceptable than emotional pain. Furthermore, women are expected to care for others rather than for themselves. These cultural factors may suggest to women that they must be physically ill before they can care for themselves. The disease model, which encourages defining physical and emotional changes as illnesses, reinforces this perspective. The program at the psychiatric hospital offers women an alternative to the traditional disease model of treatment.

PMS is experienced by women as a group of symptoms or changes that regularly occur approximately 1 week before menstruation, but are absent at other times of the month. Both physical and emotional symptoms can be experienced, such as negative affect, irritability, tiredness, food cravings, fluid retention, and headaches. As founders of the PMS Treatment Program, we were equally intent on not perpetuating the victimization of women by implying their problems were "all in their head." This was a particular danger since we work in a psychiatric hospital. We chose to focus on the relations among physical, emotional, and behavioral changes as a treatment approach. This approach validates the strengths women acquire in adapting to monthly changes in a society that offers reproduction-related options and consequences. We emphasize the positive aspects of being vulnerable to emotions premenstrually. Defining those emotions can lead to a better understanding of oneself and may be the first step in a slow evolution enabling women to use monthly emotional and behavioral changes for self-growth.

THE PROGRAM ITSELF

Assessment of each woman entering the PMS Treatment Program begins with an evaluation of the woman's understanding of the normal menstrual cycle. This is followed by an assessment of the problems that may cause premenstrual changes to reach the level of symptoms of dysfunction and an attempt to distinguish these from emotional and physical problems that exist independently from, but may be exacerbated by, premenstrual changes. Emphasis is placed on the belief that women can take responsibility for self-care if they understand the need for it.

Each of the five women therapists in the PMS Treatment Program has a commitment to working with women clients and an extensive professional history of such work with individuals and groups. Educational background is at the master's degree level or beyond in a mental health discipline (nursing, social work, counseling) and each has a minimum of 3 years of clinical experience. These multidisciplinary backgrounds, combined with the shared conviction that societal factors must be considered in working with our women clients, form a primary strength of our program.

The setting for the PMS Treatment Program provides a wide range of mental health and chemical dependency services, including couple and family therapy, inpatient treatment, and medication for the severely incapacitated. The Outpatient and Community Services Center female Medical Director shares the woman-centered, bio-psycho-social philosophy, evaluates all clients, and provides consultation to the PMS Treatment Program therapists. A gynecological consultant provides medical evaluation and follow-up when needed. Although it has been our experience that medical treatment alone, including the use of hormones or diuretics, does not reduce the severity of premenstrual symptoms on a long-term basis, gynecological treatment is made available when needed.

THE INTAKE PROCESS

Clients may be self-referred or referred by professionals in the community. Each client is contacted within 24 h and an appointment is made for the initial evaluation. This appointment takes place within 1 week of the initial contact, is the entry point to the system, and serves the following purposes:

1 Identifying presenting symptoms to determine whether they are cyclic in nature—appearing after ovulation and ceasing with the onset of menses.

2 Assessing past and present life stressors and coping skills.

3 Obtaining an accurate menstrual history encompassing the client's view of herself as a sexual, reproductive being; first impressions of menstruation; individual physiologic experiences of menses; and a sexual history.

4 Providing a thorough psycho-social history including developmental, familial, medical, vocational, and recreational dimensions.

5 Presenting natural treatment approaches, including nutritional changes, physical exercise, and relaxation techniques.

6 Explaining the importance and process of charting premenstrual symptoms.

7 Determining appropriateness of referral for gynecological exam and/or evaluation for medication.

8 Determining appropriateness of referral for psychiatric evaluation.

9 Determining appropriateness of recommending individual or group psychotherapy.

Considerable emphasis is placed on assessing the client's feelings about being a woman in a society that gives conflicting and negative messages about menstruation and choices about pregnancy. Current and original family histories often reveal roots of particularly intense emotional conflicts in these areas. Growing up in an alcoholic family system, being a survivor of incest, having been emotionally or physically abandoned by one or both parents, or experiencing a conflictual partner relationship are among the many negative experiences conducive to particular vulnerability.

Assessment tools include a Milwaukee Psychiatric Hospital Outpatient Assessment Form, a premenstrual assessment form developed by our program team and called the Daily Rating Form, and the Premenstrual Assessment Form (Halbreich, Endicott, Schacht, & Nee, 1982).

EDUCATION AND THERAPY

The educational component of our program begins during the initial evaluation. In addition to the assessment tools listed previously, a packet of materials is given to the client that includes our program philosophy with natural and recommended treatment methods, a symptom questionnaire, a daily symptom chart, a stress rating scale, and a bibliography.

After the evaluation, women may choose to work in individual or group therapy. We currently offer two PMS therapy groups, one during the day and one in the evening. Two female therapists co-facilitate each group. Each client, whether she chooses individual or group therapy, must make a 3-month commitment to our program; most clients stay from 6–12 months. The educational component of helping clients learn what is happening to their bodies and how to manage premenstrual changes continues and proceeds in conjunction with psychotherapeutic elements.

Clients are advised to make nutritional changes from time of ovulation until menses. Elimination of caffeine, salt, sugar, chocolate, and alcohol is vital. These chemical substances precipitate significant alterations in blood sugar levels, in fluid balance, and in level of consciousness, which worsen PMS symptomatology (Budoff, 1980; Lark, 1984). Six small meals of complex carbohydrates and reduced protein should be initiated to keep the blood sugar level stable. Vitamin supplements are recommended: a daily intake of a stress formula vitamin. During the premenstruum, additional Vitamin B_6, 50 mg twice a day, is suggested (Lark, 1984; Norris & Sullivan, 1984).

The importance of consistent, but not necessarily strenuous, aerobic physical activity is stressed. This promotes physical stamina, improves the oxygen delivery system, increases the blood flow to all muscles, and allows the women free time. Such activities include walking, cycling, running, swimming, yoga, and rhythmic dancing.

Recommendation of daily relaxation techniques has been included, based on recent literature (Lark, 1984) and 10 years of experience with biofeedback by one of the authors. These techniques promote utilization of alpha level awareness, allowing the body to return to a less stressful state by interfering with constant messages to maintain sympathetic nervous system responses (the stress response). These techniques include imagery, meditation, and biofeedback.

To assist a woman in gaining an awareness of her own individualized process, therapy focuses on:

1 Identifying menstrual cycle changes.
2 Evaluating stressors and stress responses and their relation to PMS symptoms.
3 Defining emotional themes in a woman's life.

4 Developing and maintaining an active and self-enhancing relationship with biological and emotional rhythms.

To clearly identify cycle changes, each woman is encouraged to closely monitor physical and emotional body signals by daily charting. Women report an awareness not only of "symptoms" that they may regard as negative or troublesome, but also of cyclic changes in personal sensitivity, which they view as positive and creative. Often, this is the first time in a woman's life that she has experienced support for attending to and valuing her biological and behavioral rhythms.

Clients are encouraged to evaluate the effect of life stress on their premenstrual symptoms. They begin to identify stressors related to cultural, biological, and personal roles as a woman. These include emotional themes, current and remote, which may surface as emotional "problems" premenstrually. Finally, women are encouraged to take an active and responsible role not only in the treatment of PMS, but also in the ongoing process of growth and change throughout the life cycle (e.g., making decisions based on personal needs, assertive communication of goals, setting limits, and accepting the wisdom that evolves with maturity). This process is particularly powerful when it occurs within the group context. There, a woman may share personal understandings, experiment with proactive behaviors, and exchange ideas and experiences in an atmosphere of support and protection. She learns that other women share many of her experiences. She no longer feels isolated.

Ruth is a good example of this group process. She is a 34-year-old, married nurse who complained of fatigue, restlessness, sadness, various physical aches and pains, abdominal bloating, headaches, and irritability—especially with her husband and two small children. She entered the program for an evaluation after 2 years of attempting to stop what she called "this emotional roller coaster." Ruth knew her marriage was suffering; she felt overwhelmed and anxious at work. She was beginning to think of herself as a "bad mother" because she was tense and angry with her children.

After an initial evaluation, Ruth was given natural treatment suggestions, was encouraged to chart symptoms daily, and was scheduled for a group that she gladly began attending. From the first, she reported feeling relief at hearing the stories of others—so similar to her own. The daily symptom charting helped her to define symptom patterns, predict times of the month that had the potential to be difficult, and arrange her busy schedule accordingly. The group treatment provided Ruth with information about the positive component of the PMS experience. The premenstrual time seemed to be a good one for feeling and identifying emotional states, really enjoying a good book, or working on a creative project. With group support, Ruth began to identify stressors in her life and ongoing emotional themes. She was able to see their relationship to PMS symptoms and to work on resolving these broader issues.

Increasingly, Ruth developed a respect for herself and for her biological and emotional rhythms. She noticed and validated changes she experienced throughout the month—moving with them, rather than against them. Ruth now reports that she knows herself and experiences herself more clearly than she did before. Her self-esteem also has improved.

In our program, we find two critical points in the therapeutic process. Those women who have dropped out of the program have generally done so at one of these turning points. The first occurs when the client begins to define the underlying painful feelings exacerbated premenstrually; the second is the moments at which life changes, which are necessary for the resolution of painful problems, need to be made. Consequences of leaving a partner, evaluating life goals, and/or redefining the role as a woman are frightening changes. Approximately 2% of women who drop out return to our programs at a later time.

FOLLOW-UP

We have begun using a posttreatment evaluation form mailed to clients at 6 months and 2 years after treatment. Before the introduction of this questionnaire, we were only able to determine the long-term results of our treatment program by voluntary self-report from clients' letters, phone calls, and group reunions.

SOME STATISTICS

Although our program is geared toward treatment rather than research, we are attempting to gather some statistical data. In the last 6 months, women receiving services at Milwaukee Psychiatric Hospital (but not necessarily candidates for our PMS Treatment Program) have been asked to complete a health and menstrual history questionnaire including the premenstrual symptom checklist. At the time of this writing, results of 66 questionnaires have been tabulated. Of the 66 forms, 18 were from women in the inpatient setting (6 of whom were in the premenstrual phase at admission); 48 were outpatients. The age range was 14 to 50 years; median age was 35 years.

Only 6 women checked "no" when asked whether they ever experienced any of 10 symptoms premenstrually. All 60 women who answered "yes" to this question identified no less than 3 symptoms. The symptoms and number of women identifying them were as follows:

Tension	53
Irritability	47
Abdominal bloating	43
Cravings for chocolate, caffeine, sugar, salt, alcohol	42
Binges (for above)	42
Fatigue	38

Water retention	37
Depression	34
Headaches	25
Suicidal thoughts	14

Of the 66 women, 30(45%) indicated they had never been pregnant. Of the 36 women with at least one pregnancy, 72% said they had experienced depression following childbirth.

Additionally, 37(56%) identified a history of emotional or mental illness in the present family and family of origin. Alcohol and/or drug dependence existed in the present family and the family of origin in 48(73%) of the 66 women.

CONCLUSION

Women experiencing premenstrual symptoms need careful evaluation by professionals competent to differentiate between premenstrual changes, premenstrual symptoms, and the presence of emotional illness. These same professionals must be equally competent to assist women not only with those issues directly related to PMS, but with the wider intrapsychic, interpersonal, and cultural contexts within which the individual woman's premenstrual experience occurs.

PMS occurs not as an isolated physiologic experience but in a living woman with her own history, psychological processes, interpersonal relationships, and lifestyle. This woman, in turn, lives not as an isolated individual or merely as a member of certain familial or nonfamilial groups, but rather as a member of a larger society, an international community of women. Had the experiences of women been different, would we simply be "treating" PMS, or rather would we be delighting in our experiences of individuality, cyclicity, and rebirth?

REFERENCES

Asso, D. (1983). *The real menstrual cycle.* New York: John Wiley and Sons.

Budoff, P. W. (1980). *No more menstrual cramps and other good news.* New York: Putnam.

Halbreich, U., Endicott, J., Schacht, S., & Nee, J. (1982). The diversity of premenstrual changes as reflected in the Premenstrual Assessment Form. *Acta Psychiatrica Scandinavica, 65,* 46–65.

Lark, S. (1984). *Premenstrual syndrome: Self-help book.* Los Altos, CA: PMS Self-Help Center.

Lever, J., & Brush, M. (1981). *Premenstrual tension.* New York: McGraw-Hill.

Norris, R. V., & Sullivan, C. (1984). *PMS: Premenstrual syndrome.* New York: Berkley Press.

SUGGESTED ADDITIONAL READINGS

Abplanalp, J. M. (1983). Psychologic components of the premenstrual syndrome: Evaluating the research and choosing the treatment. *Journal of Reproductive Medicine, 28,* 517.

Abramowitz, E., Baker, H., & Fleischer, S. (1982). Onset of depressive psychiatric crisis and the menstrual cycle. *American Journal of Psychiatry, 139,* 4.

Bender, S., & Reller, K. (1986). *PMS: A positive program to gain control.* Los Angeles, CA: Body Press.

Dalton, K. (1980). *Depression after childbirth.* New York: University Press.

Dalton, K. (1979). *Once a month.* Pomona, CA: Huner House.

Debrovner, C. H. (1983). Premenstrual syndrome. *Medical Aspects of Human Sexuality, 17*(4), 215–226.

Debrovner, C. H. (1982). *Premenstrual tension—a multidisciplinary approach.* New York: Human Sciences Press.

Dickstein, L. J. (1984). Menstrual disorders and stress in university students. *Psychiatric Annals, 14*(6), 436–441.

Eagan, A. (1983, October). The selling of premenstrual syndrome. *Ms,* pp. 27–31.

Garfinkel, P. (1984). Menstrual disorders and anorexia nervosa. *Psychiatric Annals, 14*(6), 442–446.

Gold, J. H. (1984). Menstrual disorders: Implications for clinical psychiatry. *Psychiatric Annals, 14*(6), 424–425.

Golub, S. (1983). *Lifting the curse of menstruation.* New York: Haworth Press.

Halbreich, U., & Endicott, J. (1985). Methodological issues in studies of premenstrual changes. *Psychoneuroendrocrinology, 10*(1), 15–32.

Halbreich, U., & Endicott, J. (1983). Premenstrual depressive changes. *Archives of Neurological Psychiatry, 40,* 535.

Hamilton, J., Perry, B., Alagna, S., Blumenthal, S., & Herz, E. (1984). Premenstrual mood changes: A guide to evaluation and treatment. *Psychiatric Annals, 14*(6), 426–435.

Harrison, M. (1984). *Self-help for premenstrual syndrome.* New York: Forman Publishing.

Hopson, J., & Rosenfeld, A. (1984, August). PMS: Puzzling monthly symptoms. *Psychology Today, 18*(8), 30–35.

Horrobin, D. F. (1983). The role of essential fatty acids and prostaglandins in the premenstrual syndrome. *Journal of Reproductive Medicine, 28,* 465.

Kitziner, S. (1985). *Women's experience of sex.* New York: Penguin Books.

Kraus, M., & Redman, E. (1986). Postpartum depression: An interactional view. *Journal of Marital and Family Therapy, 12*(1), 63–74.

Labrum, A. H. (1983). Hypothalamic, pineal, and pituitary factors in the premenstrual syndrome. *Journal of Reproductive Medicine, 28,* 438.

Lauerson, N., & Stukane, E. (1983). *Premenstrual syndrome and you.* New York: Simon & Schuster.

London, R. S., Sundaram, J. S., Murphy, L., & Goldstein, P. J. (1983). Evaluation and treatment of breast symptoms in patients with premenstrual syndrome. *Journal of Reproductive Medicine, 28*(8), 503–508.

Nazzaro, A., & Lombard, D. (1985). *The PMS solution.* Minneapolis, MN: Winston Press.

Osofsky, H., & Blumenthal, S. (Eds.) (1985). *Premenstrual syndrome: Current findings and future directions.* Washington, DC: American Psychiatric Press.

Paige, K. (1973, September). Women learning to sing the menstrual blues. *Psychology Today, 7*(4), 41–46.

Chapter 14

Pain Sensitivity in Dysmenorrheic and Nondysmenorrheic Women as a Function of Menstrual Cycle Phase

Eleni G. Hapidou and Denys deCatanzaro

INTRODUCTION

Dysmenorrhea, or painful menstruation, is a common gynecological condition affecting more than half of all women (Ylikorkala & Darwood, 1978). The present study employed the cold pressor task to investigate pain reactions in women with and without dysmenorrhea.

Previous studies have shown that among normally menstruating women, pain reactions vary according to cycle phase. Two studies (Goolkasian, 1980; Procacci, Zoppi, Manesca, & Romano, 1974) examined pain thresholds to radiant heat stimuli and found cyclical effects in normally menstruating women but not in oral contraceptive users or men. Procacci et al. (1974) found low threshold values during the luteal phase with a subsequent steady rise, which reached a peak toward the end of menstruation. In using signal detection to separate sensory factors from response criteria, Goolkasian (1980) found enhanced discriminability during the luteal phase but no differences in willingness to report pain according to menstrual cycle phase. However, using an aversion-to-electric-shock technique, Tedford, Warren, & Flynn (1977) obtained cyclical effects in the opposite direction: maximum sensitivity during menstruation and lowest sensitivity in the luteal phase. The differences in direction of effects have been attributed to the differences in the measures employed by the different investigators (Goolkasian, 1980).

None of these studies took into account the presence or absence of dysmenorrhea in the subjects. Very few published studies have examined pain reactions in dysmenorrheic women. As early as 1944, Haman (1944), using a pressure stimulus to induce pain on the thumb, found that dysmenorrheic women had lower thresholds than did nondysmenorrheic women, menopausal women, and men, although no statistics were reported. Goolkasian (1983), again using signal detection methods, found a significant interaction between menstrual phase and the presence or absence of dysmenorrhea. Replicating her previous findings, maximum discriminability was found in the luteal phase, but only for the nondysmenorrheic women. However, dysmenorrheic women were shown to be stable in their pain sensitivity across the menstrual cycle.

The purpose of this study was to investigate responsiveness to laboratory-induced pain in dysmenorrheic and nondysmenorrheic women over the course of the menstrual cycle. The cold pressor test was chosen as the technique of pain induction because it causes pain that resembles clinical pain in the types of sensations produced and length of tolerance (Clark & Hunt, 1971; Turk, Meichenbaum, & Genest, 1983). Thus, this study introduced an improvement over previous studies in that it employed a technique of pain induction that is comparable to that of clinical conditions. Another improvement over previous studies is that multiple dependent variables of pain assessment were employed. Whereas all the previous studies employed only assessment of pain threshold, this study also employed measures of pain tolerance and subjective pain ratings.

This study was also designed to examine psychological variables such as pain tolerance and subject pain reports in light of the adaptation-levels model (Rollman, 1979) or the hypervigilance model (Chapman, 1978). According to the former model, dysmenorrheic women should "anchor" their pain judgments according to their menstrual pain. In doing so, they would provide more conservative judgments of cold pressor pain than would nondysmenorrheic women. According to the latter model, dysmenorrheic women should be less conservative than nondysmenorrheic women because of a general sensitization to pain owing to the recurrence of menstrual pain. Haman (1944) reported lower threshold to mechanical pressure in dysmenorrheic women whereas Goolkasian (1983) showed no difference in pain sensitivity to radiant heat between dysmenorrheic and nondysmenorrheic women.

METHODS

Subjects

Sixty-five introductory psychology students volunteered for this study for course credit. Age ranged from 18 to 34 years ($\bar{X}$ = 20.02, SD = 2.76). All subjects were administered a medical screening questionnaire at the outset of the study for two purposes: to exclude pregnant women and those suffering from cardiovascular problems, hypertension, epilepsy, and fainting history, and to obtain information on menstrual cycle length and regularity and the incidence of dysmenorrhea. All menstrual cycle-related questions were "hidden" among other health-related questions. Based on this information, the experimental sessions were scheduled to occur in the follicular and luteal phases of the menstrual cycle.

Assessment of Dysmenorrhea

Subjects were categorized as dysmenorrheic or nondysmenorrheic, according to their response to a question about the presence or absence of menstrual pain/cramps. Again, this question was included in a group of questions on the incidence of different types of pain that people usually experience (headache, low back pain, other). Women who reported mild or no pain at all associated with menstruation comprised the nondysmenorrheic group. Those reporting moderate to severe pain comprised the dysmenorrheic group. This categorization did not occur until the end of the study to minimize experimenter bias. Information about medication requirements and home remedies used to counteract dysmenorrhea was also obtained.

Menstrual Cycle Phase Definition: Hormonal Patterns Over the Cycle

The normal and regular 28-day menstrual cycle is usually divided into four phases: The menstrual phase (day 1 of menstrual onset to day 7), the follicular phase (day 8–day 14), the luteal (day 15–day 21), and the premenstrual phase (day 22–day 27) (Fielding & Bosanko, 1984; Goolkasian, 1980, 1983; Tedford et al., 1977). This division is based on patterns of the ovarian hormones estrogen (estradiol) and progesterone observed at each of the cycle phases (Abplanalp, Livingston, Rose, & Sandwich, 1977). The menstrual phase is characterized by low and stable levels of estradiol and progesterone. The follicular phase, also known as postmenstrual or preovulatory, is characterized by a striking rise and a subsequent abrupt drop of estradiol. The luteal phase, also known as intermenstrual or postovulatory, is characterized by a second peak of estradiol levels and a continuous rise of progesterone levels. The premenstrual phase, also known as late luteal, is characterized by a decrease in secretion of both ovarian hormones (Abplanalp et al., 1977).

Although no laboratory tests were conducted to verify ovulation, Metcalf (1983) has reported rates of ovulation around 65% among women 5–8 years postmenarche, the approximate age range of the subjects in this study. It therefore seemed reasonable to assume that the majority of subjects did ovulate during the study. Ovulation is thought to occur 14 days before menses based on the fact that the corpus luteum has a 2-week life span (Speroff, Glass, & Kase,

1983). The postovulatory phase is considered to be the most stable in length as compared to the preovulatory phase. Thus, time of ovulation was estimated by reverse cycle day 14, that is, counting backward from the onset of the succeeding menses (Harvey, 1987). Subjects with cycles longer than 28 days were assigned the 2–3 extra days in their preovulatory phase.

Most subjects provided approximate dates of last and next expected menses during the medical screening questionnaire as well as at the end of the study, while completing the Retrospective Symptom Scale. This combined information was used to schedule and then calculate the menstrual phase during which laboratory sessions occurred.

Apparatus

The cold pressor consisted of a $57 \times 36 \times 32$ cm insulated plastic tank, which contained ice and water. A plastic mesh screen divided the tank into one section containing crushed ice and another containing ice-free water. The water was maintained at 0–1 °C and was circulated during each immersion by means of a submersible pump. A lightweight aluminum armrest contained a microswitch, which activated an adjacent computer to record total immersion time (Figure 14-1).

Subjects received a standard set of taped instructions that included a description of possible sensations (e.g., tingling, muscle cramping, and pain) and appearance changes (e.g., discoloration of hand or arm) associated with the cold pressor test. They were instructed to report the moment at which they first felt pain and to try to keep their arm in the water for "as long as possible." Subjects were also told that they could withdraw their arm at any point if they did not wish to continue.

After a cue provided on the taped instructions, subjects lowered their dominant arm into the water, which activated the computer-controlled microswitch. Immersion was terminated at the end of 4 min for subjects who had not yet withdrawn their arm. After 3–4 min, the hand becomes numb and if the subject persists more than 6–7 min, tissue damage may result. Most studies have utilized a ceiling effect of 5 min (Ashton, Ebenezer, Golding, & Thompson, 1984; Turk et al., 1983).

Measures

Cold Pressor Pain Threshold and Tolerance and Subjective Pain Ratings Threshold measures were recorded by the experimenter through the use of a stopwatch, whereas tolerance measures were automatically recorded by the computer. Subjective pain ratings were obtained after the completion of the cold pressor test. Subjects were asked to rate the degree of pain experienced during the cold pressor by using a visual analog scale. This measure was employed to obtain a direct measure of pain intensity.

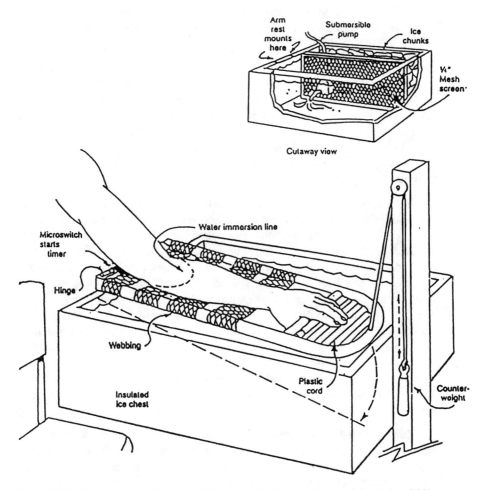

Figure 14-1   Apparatus employed in cold pressor test (adapted from Turk et al., 1983).

Visual Analog Scale   This technique, developed by Huskisson (1974), involves the use of a scale representing the continuum of the subject's experience of pain and is considered to be a very sensitive and simple method for measuring pain. The scale used in the present study was linear, horizontal, and 100 cm long. The extremes were "no pain at all" (left) and "maximum pain you can imagine" (right). A score somewhere between 0 and 100 was determined by measuring the distance from left to right. The visual analog scale (VAS) was used twice, once for rating the cold pressor pain experienced at each session and once for rating menstrual pain and overall cold pressor pain, at the end of all four experimental sessions. This comparative judgment was obtained to see how the anchoring of pain judgments (if any) occurred in the two groups.

The Pain Diary (Tursky, Tamner, & Friedman, 1982) This measure was optional. Subjects were asked to keep a daily log of hours of sleep and types and severity of pain experienced for a month beginning at the first testing session. Pain was rated as mild, moderate, or severe, to be consistent with the pain rating method of the medical screening questionnaire. These measures were taken to assess the relationship between fatigue (absence of or little sleep) and pain sensitivity and between dysmenorrhea and other types of pain. No particular types of pain were specified. It was up to each participant to record the type(s) experienced.

Retrospective Symptom Scale (RSS) (Cox & Meyer, 1978) This scale was administered once during the last session to obtain a multidimensional measure of dysmenorrhea and corroborate the initial reports of menstrual pain assessed by the medical screening questionnaire. The RSS taps physical and emotional dysmenorrheic symptoms (e.g., cramps, nausea, dizziness, irritability), medication requirements, and invalid hours (additional hours spent in bed resulting from pain). Eighteen symptoms are rated for frequency and severity on a 5-point scale according to how they were experienced in the last menstrual period. Total score is calculated as the product of frequency-severity ratings. The experimenter added a new item on menstrual cycle information. This was done to obtain the most recent menstrual onset dates. This information along with that obtained during the initial interview (medical screening questionnaire) was used to calculate the exact menstrual cycle phase during which testing occurred.

Postexperimental Questionnaire This open-ended questionnaire was devised by the experimenter for the purpose of this study. Subjects were asked to comment on their experience of the cold pressor test, to say whether they could distinguish between the cold and the painful sensation, to explain why they kept their hand in the water for as long as they did, and to provide their initial hypothesis of why the study was conducted. The primary interest was to find out whether the subjects guessed the purposes of the study.

Procedure

All volunteer subjects were administered a brief medical screening by telephone. This was done primarily to exclude subjects for whom the procedure might have presented a health risk and to obtain relevant menstrual cycle information. The subjects were told that this was a standard demographic and health information questionnaire administered in these types of investigations. Eligible subjects were then scheduled for their first experimental session corresponding to either the follicular or the luteal phase of the menstrual cycle. Both experimental sessions were scheduled for approximately the same time and day of the week. On arrival to the laboratory and before the first actual experimental session, the subjects signed an informed consent form and were given a 10-sec practice trial on the cold pressor test and then given the opportunity to withdraw. This demonstration and practice trial included a full, taped verbal description of the sensations experienced in the cold pressor and immersion of the arm into the ice water for 10 sec. Following this demonstration, the actual cold pressor test commenced. The subjects were asked to indicate the moment at which they experienced the first painful sensation (threshold) by saying "now" and to try to keep their arm in the water for as long as they could (tolerance). The cold pressor test was terminated by the experimenter after 4 min in cases where the subjects showed prolonged tolerance.

The next session was identical to the first one. The subjects were telephoned before it began to be reminded of their appointment. Following the completion of the next cold pressor session, the subjects were asked to complete the Retrospective Symptom Scale (RSS) and to rate the cold pressor pain as experienced overall, as well as their menstrual pain as experienced during the last menstrual period, on the VAS, one VAS for each type of pain. Information about onset of last menstrual period was also obtained at this time. Subjects then completed the Postexperimental Questionnaire and were debriefed.

RESULTS

Demographics

Cycle length ranged between 21 and 45 days. Acceptable cycle length ranged between 26 and 32 days. All but one of the subjects were single (98%). Two women were parous (4%). Length of menstrual flow ranged between 3 and 7 days with a mean of 4. The majority of the subjects who completed the study (70%) reported some form of menstrual pain ranging from mild to severe. Almost half of the women (44%) reported moderate to severe pain and thus comprised the dysmenorrheic group. The incidence and severity of dysmenorrhea reported in this study agree with that reported in previous studies (Hirt, Kurtz, & Ross, 1967; Stephenson, Denney, & Aberger, 1983; Wallach, 1985; Willman & White, 1986). Most dysmenorrheic women also reported the use of prescription or nonprescription prostaglandin inhibitors, oral contraceptives, or home remedies to alleviate their pain. Women using oral contraceptives were excluded from data analysis as sample size was too small to comprise a separate group ($n = 9$ with 3 exclusions). Also, the oral contraceptive users were not a homogeneous group as some were dysmenorrheic and some were not.

Subjects were asked to abstain from alcohol and analgesics for at least 10 h before each experimental session. No smokers were included in the study as smoking has been found to be associated with pain reduction (Pomerleau, Turk,

Table 14-1 **Descriptive Statistics for Cold Pressor Measures of Pain Sensitivity in the Follicular and Luteal Phase of the Cycle**

Cold pressor measures	Follicular (day 8–14)	Luteal (day 15–21)
Threshold[a]	$\bar{X}$ = 22.27	$\bar{X}$ = 16.38
	SE = 3.05	SE = 2.07
Tolerance	$\bar{X}$ = 63.12	$\bar{X}$ = 51.90
	SE = 10.19	SE = 7.44
VAS rating	$\bar{X}$ = 62.62	$\bar{X}$ = 62.89
	SE = 3.35	SE = 2.66

[a]$p < .02$.

& Fertig, 1984). Overall, exclusions because of these reasons and because of medical problems, attrition, and irregular cycles resulted in a sample of 40 subjects.

Forty normally and regularly menstruating women provided cold pressor data in the follicular and luteal phases of the cycle. Three of these subjects were excluded because of extreme tolerance scores. The remaining 37 subjects (19 dysmenorrheic and 18 nondysmenorrheic) were included in the data analysis, which utilized a 2 (group) × 2 (phase) repeated measures ANOVA, t-tests, and correlations.

Cold Pressor Pain Measures

Means and standard deviations for these three dependent measures are presented in Table 14-1.

The analysis revealed a significant phase effect for cold pressor pain threshold, F (1, 35) = 5.70, $p < .02$ (Figure 14-2). Threshold was significantly higher during the follicular ($\bar{X}$ = 22.27, SE = 3.05) as compared to the luteal phase of the cycle ($\bar{X}$ = 16.38, SE = 2.07). No other significant results were revealed through this analysis.

Significant correlations existed within the levels of the threshold measure, r (35) = .57, t = 4.14, $p < .001$; the tolerance measure, r (35) = .64, t = 4.92, $p < .001$; and the VAS measure, r (35) = .64, t = 4.98, $p < .001$.

Overall Cold Pressor Pain and Menstrual Pain Ratings

No differences were obtained for overall cold pressor pain ratings. However, group differences were found for menstrual pain ratings, F (1, 35) = 12.02, $p < .001$. The dysmenorrheic group experienced more menstrual pain during their last menstrual period ($\bar{X}$ = 47.47, SE = 5.60) than the nondysmenorrheic group ($\bar{X}$ = 21.69, SE = 4.87).

Retrospective Symptom Scale

A highly significant multivariate effect was obtained for the RSS, F (6, 30) = 3.54, p = .009 (MANOVA was performed on the RSS, the VAS, and the Total Monthly Pain Score). Significant univariate effects were obtained for menstrual symptoms, F (1, 35) = 15.88, p < .01; invalid hours, F (1, 35) = 3.99, p < .05; and medication units, F (1, 35) = 7.01, p < .001.

Significant correlations were found for all RSS measures. The more the menstrual symptoms, the more the additional hours spent in bed, r (35) = .39, t = 2.39, p < .02, and pills taken, r (35) = .32, t = 1.97, p < .05. The last two measures were also positively correlated, r (35) = .37, t = 2.33, p < .02.

RSS measures for menstrual symptoms and invalid hours were positively correlated, r (35) = .69, t = 5.57, p < .0001, and r (35) = .51, t = 3.49, p < .002, respectively. Descriptive statistics for all these measures can be seen in Table 14-2.

Pain Diary

Total Monthly Score The total monthly pain score obtained from the pain diary was calculated by summing up the products of severity ratings (mild = 1, moderate = 2, severe = 3) by each type of pain reported. For example, if a

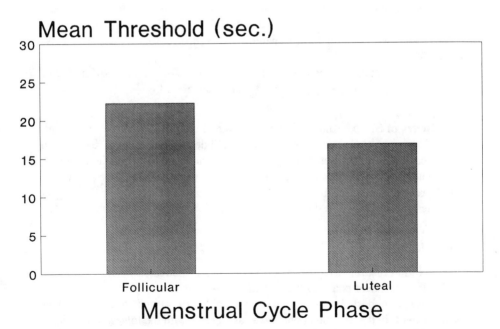

Figure 14-2 Threshold to cold pressor pain in the follicular and luteal phases of the cycle.

Table 14-2   Descriptive Statistics for Retrospective Symptom Scale (RSS) Measures, Menstrual Pain (VAS), and the Pain Diary

	Dysmenorrhea (n = 19)		Nondysmenorrhea (n = 18)	
	X̄	SE	X̄	SE
Menstrual Symptoms[a] (RSS)	46.21	6.09	13.67	2.84
Medication units[a] (RSS)	2.95	0.69	1.00	0.37
Invalid hours[a] (RSS)	2.00	0.55	0.89	0.40
Menstrual Pain[a] (VAS)	47.47	5.60	21.69	4.87
Pain diary	11.61	2.05	7.35	1.46

[a]$p < .05$.

subjects reported two types of pain with ratings of mild and moderate, the score was calculated as follows: $1 \times 1 = 1, 1 \times 2 = 2, 1 + 2 = 3$.

There were no significant differences between dysmenorrheic and nondysmenorrheic women in their monthly pain scores. However, there were significant correlations between RSS symptomatology and total monthly pain score, r (33) = .41, t = 2.58, $p < .01$ and between RSS invalid hours and total monthly pain score, r (33) = .42, t = 2.67, $p < .01$. When reports of menstrual pain/cramps were excluded from the total monthly pain score, only the RSS invalid hours measure retained the positive association with the pain score, r (33) = .34, t = 2.05, $p < .05$. Further analysis revealed that this correlation held only for the dysmenorrheic group, r (16) = .50, t = 2.29, $p < .05$.

The association between the total monthly pain score and the VAS rating of overall cold pressor pain approached significance r (33) = .32, t = 1.93, $p = .059$.

Hours of Sleep   Another measure obtained with the Pain Diary was number of hours of sleep per night. A t-test for independent samples revealed no significant differences between dysmenorrheic and nondysmenorrheic women in monthly average hours of sleep. Correlations were calculated between each cold pressor pain measure and the number of hours of sleep that the subject obtained the night before the experimental session. None were significant.

DISCUSSION

The question of cyclicity of pain sensitivity was investigated by comparing the follicular and luteal phase of the cycle in 37 women.

Results supported those of Procacci et al.'s (1974) and those of Goolkasian's (1980) in that the luteal phase was associated with the lowest threshold or maximum discriminability. However, these results only partially supported those of Goolkasian's (1983) in that no significant interaction effects were obtained in the present study. On average, both groups showed higher sensitivity (lower threshold) in the luteal phase of the cycle as compared to the follicular phase. However, inspection of the data indicates that the nondysmenorrheic group showed the largest difference between the two phases, but because of the larger variance in the follicular phase, the interaction was not significant. Perhaps with the addition of more subjects into the design, this interaction might have become significant.

These discrepancies may be also explained in terms of differences in the painful stimuli and measures employed in the two studies. Goolkasian (1980, 1983) used radiant heat stimuli, which cause cutaneous pain, whereas the present study employed the cold pressor test, which induces deep pain. The differences between these two types of pain have been discussed by Procacci (1969). In contrast to deep pain, cutaneous pain is "bright" and well localized, and it is not accompanied by autonomic reactions, such as changes in blood pressure, sweating, and nausea. Deep somatic pain, such as that induced by the cold pressor, is accompanied by autonomic reflexes such as rise in blood pressure, muscle ischemia, and irradiation of pain.

It is also possible that the discriminability measure employed by Goolkasian (1983) was sensitive enough to discriminate between the two groups in the different phases, whereas the cold pressor pain threshold was not. Moreover, Goolkasian's method of menstrual phase assignment might have been more accurate in that she employed basal body temperature charts (BBT) for determining ovulation. Even though BBT is only 80% accurate in demonstrating ovulation as compared to direct hormone assays (Moghissi, 1976), it is still more accurate than relying on the natural 65% rate of ovulation occurring in young women (Metcalf, 1983). It is possible that the large within-group variances obtained in this study were partly a result of absence of ovulation in some women. However, the logistics of this study did not allow us to employ sophisticated techniques for determining ovulation. Subjects had to remain naive to the purposes of the study, and we did not have adequate financial and temporal resources to employ such techniques. Moreover, it is not at all uncommon to rely on the occurrence of normal and regular cycles to conduct studies on menstrual phase effects. A number of studies on the menstrual cycle relied on information regarding menstrual regularity and onset of most recent menses for phase definition (Kelleher, Joyce, Kelly, & Ferris, 1986; Olasov & Jackson, 1987). However, Abplanalp et al. (1977) found that this indirect method for determining ovulation is no better than chance (50%).

Some evidence exists to support these results in terms of fluctuating gonadal hormone levels. In measuring changes in breast sensitivity with two-point discrimination thresholds, Robinson and Short (1977) obtained maximal sensitivity at ovulation and at menstruation. Since no changes occurred in oral contraceptive users, the elevated pain thresholds were attributed to declining levels of hormones around menstruation and ovulation.

Kenshalo (1966) found that cool thresholds decrease in the luteal phase as compared to the follicular phase. These differences were attributed to the release of progesterone following ovulation. When progesterone derivatives were administered on the fifth day of the cycle, cool sensitivity was increased. Differences between the follicular and luteal phases have also been demonstrated on vibrotactile sensitivity (Gescheider, Verillo, McCann, & Aldrich, 1984). Lower thresholds to a vibrotactile stimulus of 250 Hz occurred in the luteal phase as compared to the follicular phase in normally menstruating women only. Further differences between the two phases have been demonstrated by Hastrup and Light (1984). These investigators showed that cardiovascular responsiveness to a reaction time task was higher in the luteal than in the follicular phase. Presence of estrogen and progesterone during the luteal phase was implicated for increasing cardiac output since combined estrogen/progestin oral contraceptives are known to increase blood volume, stroke volume, and cardiac output (Lehtovirts, 1974).

All these studies point to the validity of cyclicity of a variety of effects over the course of the menstrual cycle and further demonstrate that explanation in terms of gonadal hormone fluctuations is tenable. However, these conclusions are tentative unless such effects are corroborated by direct measurements of hormonal levels.

Although significant correlations were found between pain threshold and tolerance, no phase differences in tolerance were obtained. Tolerance is considered to be a learned component of pain, mostly related to ethnic, cultural, psychological, and situational factors (Ahles, Blanchard, & Leventhal, 1983; Bandura, O'Leary, Barr-Taylor, Gauthier, & Gossard, 1987; Clark, 1969; Gelfand, 1964; Friedman, Thompson, & Rosen, 1985; Lambert, Libman, & Poser, 1960; Tursky, 1973; Weisenberg, Kreindler, Schachat, & Werboff, 1975; Wolff, Krasnegor, & Farr, 1965). Threshold is considered to be an unlearned component, mostly dependent on physiological variables (Gelfand, 1964; Wolff et al., 1965; Wolff & Horland, 1967). The fact that only threshold varies across menstrual phase may indicate that, as a sensory phenomenon, threshold is influenced by the hormonal changes occurring around ovulation.

The tolerance measure, with its psychological and motivational components, failed to discriminate between the two groups. It has been the implicit assumption of clinicians and gynecologists that dysmenorrheic women differ from nondysmenorrheic women in nonsensory factors such as attitudes toward menstruation and the feminine role (Cox & Meyer, 1978; Levitt & Lubin, 1967). The tolerance measure was used in this study to allow such psychological differences between these two groups to emerge. However, tolerance was correlated with threshold, and did not discriminate between the two groups in any of the phases. If anything, the tolerance measure was also quite variable and skewed. Also, Aberger, Denney, & Hutchings (1983) and Ashton et al. (1984) obtained tolerance data that were highly variable and skewed to the right.

In general, this study found that the cold pressor test did not discriminate between women who reported pain associated with menstruation and those with relatively pain-free menstrual periods. Cold pressor pain was assessed using threshold, tolerance, and subjective ratings (VAS). Dysmenorrheic and nondysmenorrheic women did not differ significantly on any of these measures. Similar findings have also been reported by Aberger et al. (1983), who employed an ischemic pain procedure to measure pain threshold, tolerance, and subjective pain ratings in different groups of dysmenorrheic women. Results from both studies are also in agreement with those reported by Cox and Meyer (1978).

Reports of dysmenorrhea, as assessed according to the subject's responses during the medical screening questionnaire, were validated by the RSS measures and the VAS rating of menstrual pain (Cox & Meyer, 1978). Dysmenorrheic women experienced significantly more frequent and severe menstrual symptoms, used more medications, spent more hours in bed, and rated their menstrual pain higher than did nondysmenorrheic women. The VAS has also been found to be a valid measure in the evaluation of premenstrual symptoms (Casper & Powell, 1986; Rubinow, Roy-Byrne, Hoban, Gold, & Post, 1984) and in various types of chronic pain (Beery & Huskisson, 1972; Huskisson, 1974; Joyce, Zutshi, Hrubes, & Mason, 1975; McGuire, 1984; Ohnhaus & Adler, 1975; Price, McGrath, Rafii, & Buckingham, 1983; Scott & Huskisson, 1976; Woodforde & Merskey, 1971).

Postexperimental questionnaire data provided by the two groups of subjects were treated as anecdotal information and used to further support the general lack of difference between the groups and the view that tolerance depends on psychological factors. Both the dysmenorrheic and nondysmenorrheic groups included subjects who reached maximum levels of tolerance, and both groups had subjects who reported the use of distraction techniques or viewed the cold pressor test as a challenge for demonstrating "self control" and "strength." In commenting about their various motives for tolerating pain, a few women said that they would tolerate a lot of pain if that meant saving their children's or their own lives. However, for a psychology experiment, even if that meant course credit, they were not willing to tolerate a lot of pain. This and other similar comments only reinforce the commonly held view that pain tolerance is more a psychological than a physiological phenomenon. As such, pain tolerance represents the reactive or emotional component of pain that includes emotional reactions to and fearful expectations about the pain experience (Beecher, 1969; Tursky, 1973). Although largely anecdotal, these findings support those of Aberger et al. (1983), who found no cognitive and behavioral coping strategy differences between dysmenorrheic and nondysmenorrheic women.

The two groups did not differ in their overall experience of pain during the month as shown by their pain diary scores. No significant differences were obtained between the two groups. Nondysmenorrheic women were as likely or unlikely as dysmenorrheic women to report different kinds of pain (mostly headaches, stomachaches, sinus pain, and sports-related pain) during the month. Because the study was conducted in the winter, and around midterm exams, a number of subjects reported sinus pain from colds and stomachaches "resulting from stress" (their interpretation). However, some interesting correlations did emerge from the data. The total monthly pain score was correlated with the VAS rating of overall cold pressor pain, that is, the higher the reported incidence of pain during the month, the higher the degree of pain as experienced in the cold pressor test. This correlation approached significance. Since no between-group differences were obtained, this result may indicate a general tendency of subjects for reacting to pain. This, in turn, supports a hypervigilance or sensitization model of pain judgment. However, this does not apply to dysmenorrhea. A finding obtained relevant to dysmenorrhea was that of a positive correlation between the total monthly pain score and the RSS measure of invalid hours. This may indicate a general tendency of subjects who report more pain during the month to also spend additional time in bed because of menstrual discomfort. This result held only for dysmenorrheic subjects even after reports of menstrual pain were excluded from the monthly pain score. These findings point to patterns of "illness behaviors" (Mechanic, 1962).

No significant between-group differences were obtained in average number of hours of sleep during the month or within the two menstrual phases. Moreover, number of hours of sleep was not significantly correlated with either measure of cold pressor pain. Sleep in the two menstrual phases was not significantly different from the average monthly sleep.

Pain judgment in dysmenorrhea, as investigated in this study, does not lend itself to interpretation in terms of the adaptation levels model (Rollman, 1979) or the hypervigilance model (Chapman, 1978). Dysmenorrheic women were neither less sensitive nor more sensitive than nondysmenorrheic women in their experience of cold pressor pain. The data would fit the hypervigilance model had the dysmenorrheic women shown higher sensitivity than nondysmenorrheic women. This would also have supported the view that dysmenorrhea, as a pain phenomenon, has psychogenic origins. However, with the discovery of prostaglandins, as an important etiological factor of dysmenorrhea, it has become more difficult to argue in favor of psychogenic origins (Rauh, Lucas, Shepherd, & Burket, 1985). The data would fit the adaptation-levels model had the dysmenorrheic women shown lower sensitivity than the nondysmenorrheic women and/or provided more conservative judgments of cold pressor pain. The only trend in the data pointing to that direction was obtained with the subjective ratings of cold pressor pain. Dysmenorrheic women tended to provide lower VAS ratings than nondysmenorrheic women. However, even though this measure was the least variable of the three cold pressor measures, no significant results were obtained. This tendency, if any, disappeared when the subjects were asked to provide an overall measure of cold pressor pain at the end of all sessions. This may be a result of the fact that in this instance, subjects used the cold pressor pain (intense and most recent experience) as the comparison point for rating their menstrual pain. This tendency for lower pain ratings in dysmenorrheic women was further investigated in a later study in this laboratory, which will be reported later.

REFERENCES

Aberger, W. W., Denney, D. R., & Hutchings, D. F. (1977). Pain sensitivity and coping strategies among dysmenorrheic women: Much ado about nothing. *Behavior Research Theory, 21,* 119–127.

Abplanalp, T. W., Livingston, L., Rose, R. M., & Sandwich, D. (1977). Cortisol and growth hormone response to psychological stress during the menstrual cycle. *Psychosomatic Medicine, 39,* 158–177.

Ahles, T. A., Blanchard, E. B., & Leventhal, H. (1983). Cognitive control of pain: Attention to the sensory aspects of the cold pressor stimulus. *Cognitive Therapy and Research, 7*(2), 159–178.

Ashton, H., Ebenezer, I., Golding, J. F., & Thompson, J. W. (1984). Effects of acupuncture and transcutaneous electrical nerve stimulation on cold-induced pain in normal subjects. *Journal of Psychosomatic Research, 28*(4), 301–308.

Bandura, A., O'Leary, A., Barr-Taylor, C., Gauthier, J., & Gossard, D. (1987). Perceived self-efficacy and pain control: Opioid and nonopioid mechanisms. *Journal of Personality and Social Psychology, 53*(3), 563–571.

Beecher, H. K. (1959). *Measurement of subjective responses.* New York: Oxford University Press.

Beery, H., & Huskisson, E. C. (1972). Measurement of pain. *Journal of Clinical Trials, 9,* 13–18.

Casper, R. F., & Powell, A. M. (1986). Premenstrual syndrome: Documentation by a linear analog scale compared with two descriptive scales. *American Journal of Obstetrics and Gynecology, 155*(4), 862–867.

Chapman, C. R. (1978). The perception of noxious events. In R. A. Sternbach (Ed.), *The psychology of pain.* New York: Raven Press.

Clark, W. C. (1969). Sensory-decision theory analysis of the placebo effect on the criterion pain and thermal sensitivity. *Journal of Abnormal Psychology, 74,* 363–371.

Clark, W. C., & Hunt, H. F. (1971). Pain. In J. A. Downey & R. C. Darling (Eds.), *Physiological basis for rehabilitation medicine.* Philadelphia: W. B. Saunders.

Cox, D. J., & Meyer, R. G. (1978). Behavioral treatment parameters with primary dysmenorrhea. *Journal of Behavioral Medicine, 1,* 297–310.

Fielding, D., & Bosanko, C. (1984). Psychological aspects of the menstruum and premenstruum. In A. Broome & L. Wallace (Eds.), *Psychology and gynecological problems* (pp. 211–242). London: Tavistock Publications.

Friedman, H., Thompson, R. B., & Rosen, E. F. (1985). Perceived threat as a major factor in tolerance for experimentally induced cold-water pain. *Journal of Abnormal Psychology, 94*(4), 624–629.

Gelfand, S. (1964). The relationship of experimental pain tolerance to pain threshold. *Canadian Journal of Psychology, 18,* 36–41.

Gescheider, G. A., Verillo, R. T., McCann, J. T., & Aldrich, E. M. (1984). Effects of the menstrual cycle of vibrotactile sensitivity. *Perception and Psychophysics, 36*(6), 586–592.

Goolkasian, P. (1980). Cyclic changes in pain perception: An ROC analysis. *Perception and Psychophysics, 27,* 499–504.

Goolkasian, P. (1983). An ROC analysis of pain reactions in dysmenorrheic and non-dysmenorrheic women. *Perception and Psychophysics, 34*(4), 381–386.

Haman, J. O. (1944). Pain threshold in dysmenorrhea. *American Journal of Obstetrics and Gynecology, 47,* 686–691.

Harvey, S. M. (1987). Female sexual behavior: Fluctuations during the menstrual cycle. *Journal of Psychosomatic Research, 31*(1), 101–110.

Hastrup, J. L., & Light, K. C. (1984). Sex differences in cardiovascular stress responses: Modulation as a function of menstrual cycle phases. *Journal of Psychosomatic Research, 28*(6), 475–483.

Hirt, M., Kurtz, R., & Ross, W. D. (1967). The relationship between dysmenorrhea and selected personality variables. *Psychosomatics, 8,* 350.

Huskisson, E. C. (1974). Measurement of pain. *Lancet, ii,* 1127–1131.

Joyce, C. R. B., Zutshi, D. W., Hrubes, V., & Mason, R. M. (1975). Comparison of fixed interval and visual analogue scales for rating chronic pain. *European Journal of Clinical Pharmacology, 8,* 415–420.

Kelleher, C., Joyce, C., Kelly, G., & Ferris, J. B. (1986). Blood pressure alters during the normal menstrual cycle. *British Journal of Obstetrics & Gynecology, 93*(5), 523–526.

Kenshalo, D. R. (1966). The cool threshold associated with phases of the menstrual cycle. *Journal of Applied Physiology, 21,* 1031–1039.

Lambert, J. P., Libman, E., & Poser, E. G. (1960). *Journal of Personality, 38,* 350–357.

Lehtovirts, W. (1974). Haemodynamic effects of combined estrogen/progestogen oral contraceptives. *Journal of Obstetrics and Gynecology of British Commonwealth, 81,* 517–525.

Levitt, E. E., & Lubin, B. (1967). Some personality factors associated with menstrual complaints and menstrual attitude. *Journal of Psychosomatic Research, 21,* 267–270.

McGuire, D. B. (1984). The measurement of clinical pain. *Nursing Research, 33,* 152–156.

Mechanic, D. (1962). The concept of illness behavior. *Journal of Chronic Disease, 15,* 189–194.

Metcalf, M. (1983). Incidence of ovulation from the menarche to the menopause: Observations of 622 New Zealand women. *New Zealand Medical Journal, 96,* 645–648.

Moghissi, K. S. (1976). Accuracy of basal body temperature for ovulation detection. *Fertility and Sterility, 27,* 1415–1421.

Ohnhaus, E., & Adler, R. (1975). Methodological problems in the measurement of pain: A comparison between the verbal rating scale and the visual analogue scale. *Pain, 1,* 379–384.

Olasov, B., & Jackson, J. (1987). Effects of expectancies on women's reports of moods during the menstrual cycle. *Psychosomatic Medicine, 49*(1), 65–77.

Pomerleau, O. F., Turk, D. C., & Fertig, J. B. (1984). The effects of cigarette smoking on pain and anxiety. *Addictive Behaviors, 9*(3), 265–271.

Price, D. D., McGrath, P. A., Rafii, A., & Buckingham, B. (1983). The validation of visual analogue scales as ratio scale measures for chronic and experimental pain. *Pain, 17,* 45–56.

Procacci, P. (1969). A survey of modern concepts of pain. In P. J. Vinken, & G. W. Bruyn (Eds.), *Handbook of clinical neurology* (vol. 1, pp. 114–146). Amsterdam: North-Holland.

Procacci, P., Zoppi, M., Manesca, M., & Romano, S. (1974). Studies of the pain threshold in man. In J. R. Green & R. A. Thompson (Eds.), *Advances in neurology* (vol. 4) New York: Raven Press.

Rauh, T. L., Lucas, P., Shepherd, T., & Burket, R. (1985). Dysmenorrhea in adolescence. *Medical Aspects of Human Sexuality, 19*(1), 134–155.

Robinson, J. E., & Short, R. V. (1977) Changes in breast sensitivity at puberty, during the menstrual cycle, and at parturition. *British Medical Journal, 1,* 118–1191.

Rollman, G. B. (1979). Signal detection theory pain measures: Empirical validation studies and adaptation-level effects. *Pain, 6,* 9–21.

Rubinow, B., Roy-Byrne, P., Hoban, M., Gold, P., & Post, R. (1984). Prospective assessment of menstrually related mood disorders. *American Journal of Psychiatry, 141,* 664–686.

Scott, J., & Huskisson, E. C. (1976). Graphic representation of pain. *Pain, 2*(2), 175–184.

Speroff, L., Glass, R. H., & Kase, N. G. (1983). *Clinical gynecologic endocrinology and infertility.* Baltimore, MD: Williams & Wilkins.

Stephenson, L. A., Denney, D. R., & Aberger, E. W. (1983). Factor structure of the menstrual symptom questionnaire relationship to oral contraceptives, neuroticism, and life stress. *Behavior Research and Therapy, 21,* 129–135.

Tedford, W. H., Warren, D. E., & Flynn, W. E. (1977). Alteration of shock aversion thresholds during the menstrual cycle. *Perception and Psychophysics, 21,* 193–196.

Turk, D. C., Meichenbaum, D., & Genest, M. (1983). *Pain and behavioral medicine. A cognitive perspective.* New York: Guilford Press.

Tursky, B. (1973). Physical, physiological, and psychological factors that affect pain reaction to electric shock. *Psychophysiology, 11*(2), 95–112.

Tursky, B., Tamner, L. D., & Friedman, R. (1982). The pain perception profile: A psychophysical approach to the assessment of pain report. *Behavior Therapy, 13,* 376–394.

Wallach, H. (1985). *Dysmenorrhea: Prevalence and characteristics.* Paper presented at the Joint International Meeting of the Canadian Pain Society and the Intractable pain Society of Great Britain and Ireland, Halifax, August 1985.

Weisenberg, M., Kreindler, M. L., Schachat, R., & Werboff, J. (1975). Pain: Anxiety and attitudes in Black, White and Puerto Rican patients. *Psychosomatic Medicine,* *37,* 123–135.

Willman, B. G., & White, P. A. (1986). Assessment of dysmenorrhea using the menstrual symptom questionnaire: Factor structure and validity. *Behavior Research and Therapy, 24*(5), 547–551.

Wolff, B. B., & Horland, A. A. (1967). Effects of suggestion upon experimental pain: A validation study. *Journal of Abnormal Psychology, 22,* 402–407.

Wolff, B. B., Krasnegor, N. A., & Farr, R. S. (1965). Effect of suggestion upon experimental pain response parameters. *Perceptual and Motor Skills, 21,* 675–683.

Woodforde, J. M., & Merskey, H. (1971). Correlation between verbal scale and visual analogue scale and pressure algometer. *Journal of Psychosomatic Research, 16,* 173–178.

Ylikorkala, O., & Darwood, M. Y. (1978). New concepts in dysmenorrhea. *American Journal of Obstetrics and Gynecology, 130,* 833–841.

Chapter 15

A Study of Headache
Intensity and Disability
with the Menstrual Cycle

Patricia Solbach, Lolafaye Coyne, and Joseph Sargent

INTRODUCTION

Headache is a common ailment. Research in the last several decades has focused on the etiology, diagnosis, and treatment of this frequent complaint. Menstrually exacerbated headaches have only recently begun to be examined, with the focus of current work on the menstrual migraine headache (Solbach, Sargent, & Coyne, 1984; Solbach, Sargent, & Kennedy, 1986).

Many women experience headaches around their menstrual period. In a study of the prevalence of perimenstrual symptoms, Woods, Most, and Dery (1982) found a headache incidence rate greater than 30% in their sample. The study found that factors influencing the incidence rate during the menstrual phase were age, race, education, and income. Black women reported more menstrual headaches, whereas older women and those with more education and greater incomes had fewer menstrual headaches. No such variables were identified for the premenstrual phase.

Although other researchers have found similar incidence rates of 30% or more for headache in their samples (Moos, 1968; Pennington, 1957), none have

The authors thank James Taylor, PhD, for his work constructing the scales and Jimmie Gleason, MD, Ob/Gyn, for his consultation on this study.

examined in depth the nature of the menstrually exacerbated headache, which is usually of two types.

One type is the menstrual migraine headache—a one-sided, throbbing head pain usually associated with gastrointestinal upset, photophobia, and irritability (Solbach, 1985). The other type of headache is known as tension or muscle contraction headache, described as an ache or a sensation of tightness or pressure, usually in the frontal and occipital area and varying widely in frequency, duration, and intensity (Martin, 1983).

The menstrual migraine headache is thought to be influenced by the fluctuation of estrogen levels through the sympathetic nervous system (Welch, Darnley, & Simkons, 1984). The etiology of the other menstrually exacerbated headache is less certain. Whether the menstrually exacerbated tension headache, like other menstrual symptoms, is socially learned, has a psychodynamic component, or is a result of a hormonal biological basis has not been conclusively demonstrated (Dennerstein & Burrows, 1979).

The tension headache is usually less intense and disabling than the migraine headache. In assessing the qualities of tension headache pain, Hunter and Philips (1981) found that researchers have shown little interest in the subjective component of headache pain, which includes pain intensity, its sensory and emotional qualities, and pain evaluation. Hunter's headache scale, which was adopted from the McGill Pain Questionnaire, was developed to provide a better assessment of this component (Hunter, 1983). Other assessment tools have been based on analog or adjectival scales in the form of headache diaries, which vary widely in their use in headache research reports.

This study examines the menstrually exacerbated tension headache occurrence in 32 women over 9 months in which a minimum of 5 menstrual cycles were reported. Headache intensity and disability were closely monitored on example-anchored, 100-point scales and together with headache frequency and duration were evaluated to see if any differences exist between the menstrually exacerbated tension headache and tension headaches occurring at other times.

METHODS

Data for this study were gathered as part of a larger, federally funded project evaluating the effectiveness of nondrug treatments for the control of headache (Sargent, Solbach, Coyne, Spohn & Segerson, 1986; Sargent, Solbach, & Coyne, 1987). Four independent nondrug techniques were evaluated: no treatment, autogenic phrases, electromyographic biofeedback, and thermal biofeedback.

Subjects participated for 36 weeks and were required to keep daily records of headache activity. Each subject participated in 22 laboratory sessions in which hand temperature and electromyographic measurements were recorded.

The 36-week project was divided into a 4-week baseline, an 8-week training period, and a 24-week follow-up. At the end of the study, each subject underwent a debriefing interview.

Subjects with the diagnosis of tension headache were accepted into the study. Subjects underwent a complete physical and neurological exam before entering the project. Those who had severe physical or psychological problems were excluded from the study.

During the 36 weeks, subjects charted daily their headache frequency, intensity, disability, duration, symptoms, medication usage, and menses. Example-anchored, 100-point scales were used to measure headache intensity and disability (Figures 15-1 & 15-2).

The scales were constructed to provide more sensitive and accurate self-report measurements (Taylor, 1968a, 1968b; Taylor, Ptacek, Carithers, Griffin, & Coyne, 1972). Scale construction consisted of collecting a number of specific descriptors from headache patients to illustrate head pain intensity and disability. Six judges who were familiar with head pain rank-ordered the descriptors, and the agreement of the rankings was statistically evaluated.

Descriptors with consistent ranks were selected to illustrate the interval markers for each scale. Headache disability was less difficult to scale as it involved observable behavior, whereas headache intensity was more subjective.

Differences in menstruation related headaches, defined as those occurring in the 3 days before and all days during the menstrual flow, and headaches occurring at other times were examined. Comparisons using headache frequency, duration, intensity, and disability were made between the two time periods.

The method of data analysis was multivariate profile analysis with one independent factor (treatment group), with four groups, and with two correlated factors: menstrual/nonmenstrual and cycle block with five levels. Following the convention for multivariate analysis, a p value of $\leq .15$ was considered to be interpretable. Four dependent variables—headache frequency, duration, intensity, and disability—were analyzed.

RESULTS

A total of 69 females entered the project, 22 subjects dropped out of the project, 6 others had had hysterectomies, 4 more were postmenopausal, and 5 had data with less than 5 menstrual cycles. This paper reports on the 32 females who completed the study, were menstruating, and reported a minimum of 5 menstrual cycles over the 9-month study.

The average age of the sample subject was 29 years, with a range of 14 to 46 years of age. Twenty-four subjects (75%) reported a family history of headache, with 17 reporting a female line of headache sufferers.

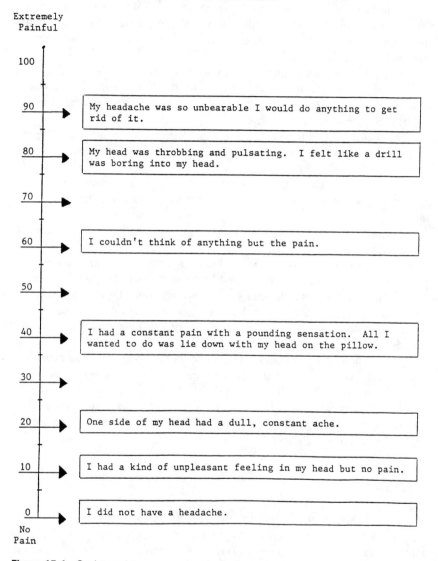

Figure 15-1   Scale used to measure headache intensity.

Disability Scale

HOW DISRUPTED OR DISABLING WAS YOUR HEADACHE TODAY?

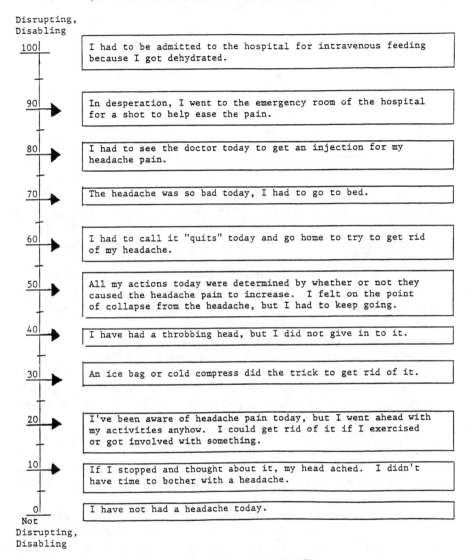

Disrupting,
Disabling

100 | I had to be admitted to the hospital for intravenous feeding because I got dehydrated.

90 | In desperation, I went to the emergency room of the hospital for a shot to help ease the pain.

80 | I had to see the doctor today to get an injection for my headache pain.

70 | The headache was so bad today, I had to go to bed.

60 | I had to call it "quits" today and go home to try to get rid of my headache.

50 | All my actions today were determined by whether or not they caused the headache pain to increase. I felt on the point of collapse from the headache, but I had to keep going.

40 | I have had a throbbing head, but I did not give in to it.

30 | An ice bag or cold compress did the trick to get rid of it.

20 | I've been aware of headache pain today, but I went ahead with my activities anyhow. I could get rid of it if I exercised or got involved with something.

10 | If I stopped and thought about it, my head ached. I didn't have time to bother with a headache.

0 | I have not had a headache today.

Not
Disrupting,
Disabling

Figure 15-2 Scale used to measure headache-related disability.

Table 15-1   Intensity Means for Menstrual and Nonmenstrual Headaches

Menstrual period	Headache type	Mean	Combined mean
1	NM	27.493	28.260
	M	29.026	
2	NM	24.968	24.042
	M	23.117	
3	NM	20.011	22.026
	M	24.040	
4	NM	20.206	20.966
	M	21.726	
5	NM	17.762	18.288
	M	18.815	

The average length of the headache problem before entry into the study was 13 years. Nineteen subjects had chronic tension headaches, defined as a minimum of 5 per week, and 13 had episodic tension headaches, defined as less than 5 headaches per week. Four were taking birth control pills during the 9 months.

Problems unique to the study were encountered in the analyses and interpretation of the data as a result of the individual differences among the subjects in menstrual patterns. Only 6 subjects started out in the project with a menstrual period; thus, their second cycle was used with the first cycle of the other 26 subjects. Each subjects' first analyzable cycle occurred in the 4-week baseline or early training period. All subjects were evaluated on 5 menstrual periods.

Statistical analysis of the data showed some differences between the menstruating and nonmenstruating headache occurrences. There were proportionately more menstrual headaches ($\bar{x} = 0.681$) than nonmenstrual headaches ($\bar{x} = 0.672$), but this was not significant. The menstrual headaches decreased significantly less across time with treatment than the nonmenstrual headaches ($F = 2.827$; $df = 4, 25$; $p < .046$). No significant difference was found in duration between menstrual and nonmenstrual headaches. Duration decreased significantly across time with treatment for both groups ($F = 2.293$; $df = 4, 25$; $p < .088$).

The menstrual headaches were found to be slightly more intense ($\bar{x} = 23.3$) than the nonmenstrual headaches ($\bar{x} = 22.1$) ($F = 1.895$; $df = 4, 25$; $p < .143$). Table 15-1 shows a higher intensity mean rating for menstrual headaches for all the menstrual periods except the second period where the intensity mean for the menstrual headaches is 23.1 and for the nonmenstrual headaches 24.9, but these are not significantly different. All subjects showed improvement in headache intensity across time with treatment for both menstrual and nonmenstrual headaches ($F = 5.650$, $df = 4, 25$; $p < .002$).

There was no significant difference in disability between the menstrual and nonmenstrual headaches. Table 15-2 shows a higher disability mean rating for menstrual headaches for all the menstrual periods except the second period where the disability mean for the menstrual headaches is 20.4 and for the nonmenstrual headaches 22.2, but these are not significantly different. All subjects showed improvement in headache disability across time with treatment for both menstrual and nonmenstrual headache ($F = 5.361$; $df = 4, 25$; $p < .003$).

Treatment outcome comparing the four groups is presented in another paper (Solbach, Sargent, Coyne, Malone, & Simons, 1988).

DISCUSSION

Results of this study show that menstrually exacerbated tension headaches are different from tension headaches occurring at other times. There are proportionately more of them, they are more intense, and they decrease less over time with treatment than tension headaches that do not occur around the menses.

Mean ratings of intensity and disability for both menstrual and nonmenstrual headaches were relatively low, with average means under 30 on a 100-point scale. This was not unexpected, since the scale means are higher for migraines and thus the scales can aid in the differential diagnosis of the two headache types.

Further examination of Tables 15-1 and 15-2 shows that the intensity and disability ratings were at similar intervals on each scale. The mean intensity of menstrual headaches for the 5 periods was 23.3. The descriptor "one side of my head had a dull, constant ache" illustrated this intensity level. The mean disability for the 5 periods was 20.9, and the descriptor illustrating this level reflected that although the subject was aware of the headache, she nevertheless pursued her activities.

Table 15-2   Disability Means for Menstrual and Nonmenstrual Headaches

Menstrual period	Headache type	Mean	Combined mean
1	NM	25.423	25.648
	M	25.872	
2	NM	22.178	21.304
	M	20.430	
3	NM	18.630	19.973
	M	21.316	
4	NM	18.249	18.968
	M	19.686	
5	NM	16.319	16.831
	M	17.345	

Higher intensity and disability levels for the menstrually exacerbated headaches were not influenced by the subjects' awareness of or expectation that they would be so, as in other studies of menstrual symptomatology. The focus of this study was treatment outcome for tension headache. Attention was not paid to menstrually exacerbated headaches other than by having subjects mark the daily record sheet if they were menstruating that day.

A shortcoming of this study was that data collection did not begin at the same point for all subjects. Preferably it should have begun with the onset of the menstrual period for each subject. Thus, data collected from different points in the study was compared. This occurred, for the most part, in the baseline phase (first 4 weeks) and in the first 2 weeks of the training phase.

The menstrually exacerbated tension headache, although rarely severe, nevertheless can be troublesome. No single drug or nondrug technique has been found universally effective for it. Subjects in this study indicated that they coped with their headaches by continuing with their activities or getting involved in something. Exercising, particularly facial exercises, can help relieve the tight, tense muscles.

More attention must be given to menstrually exacerbated headaches before effective treatments emerge. Many current sufferers will be helped simply when treatment providers acknowledge that headaches that occur around the menses are different from the rank-and-file headache and are to be understood and treated as such.

REFERENCES

Dennerstein, L., & Burrows, G. D. (1979). Affect and the menstrual cycle. *Journal of Affective Disorders, 1*, 77–92.

Hunter, M. (1983). The headache scale: A new approach to the assessment of headache pain based on pain descriptions. *Pain, 16*, 361–373.

Hunter, M., & Philips, C. (1981). The experience of headache—An assessment of the qualities of tension headache pain. *Pain, 10*, 209–219.

Martin, M. J. (1983). Muscle-contraction (tension) headache. *Psychosomatics, 24*, 319–324.

Moos, R. H. (1968). The development of a menstrual distress questionnaire. *Psychosomatic Medicine, 30*, 853–867.

Pennington, V. (1957). Meprobamate (Miltown) in premenstrual tension. *Journal of the American Medical Association, 164*, 638–640.

Sargent, J., Solbach, P., & Coyne, L. (1987, June). A controlled, experimental outcome study of non-drug treatments for tension headache. Presented to the American Association for the Study of Headache, Quebec City, Canada.

Sargent, J., Solbach, P., Coyne, L., Spohn, H., & Segerson, J. (1986). Results of a controlled, experimental, outcome study of non-drug treatments for the control of migraine headache. *Journal of Behavioral Medicine, 9*, 291–323.

Solbach, P. (1985). Menstruation: A study of menstrual migraine headache. Presented to the 6th Conference of the Society for Menstrual Cycle Research, Galveston, Texas.

Solbach, P., Sargent, J., & Coyne, L. (1984). Menstrual migraine headache: Results of a controlled, experimental, outcome study of non-drug treatments. *Headache, 24,* 75–78.

Solbach, P., Sargent, J., Coyne, L., Malone, L. & Simons, A. (1988). Tension headache: A comparison of menstrual and non-menstrual occurrences. *Headache, 28,* 108–110.

Solbach, P., Sargent, J., & Kennedy, K. (1986). Migraine headache associated with menstruation. *IM-Internal Medicine for the Specialist, 7,* 93–103.

Taylor, J. B. (1968a). Rating scales as measures of clinical judgment: A method for increasing scale reliability and sensitivity. *Educational and Psychological Measurement, 28,* 747–766.

Taylor, J. B. (1968b). A brief ranking method as an alternative to Thurstone scaling procedures. *Perceptual and Motor Skills, 16,* 533–534.

Taylor, J. B., Ptacek, M., Carithers, M., Griffin, C., & Coyne, L. (1972). Rating scales as measures of clinical judgment. III. Judgments of the self on personality inventories and direct ratings. *Educational and Psychological Measurement, 32,* 543–557.

Welch, K. M. A., Darnley, D., & Simkons, R. (1984). The role of estrogen in migraine: A review and hypothesis. *Cephalalgia, 4,* 227–236.

Woods, N. F., Most, A., & Dery, G. K. (1982). Prevalence of premenstrual symptoms. *American Journal of Public Health, 72,* 1257–1264.

Chapter 16

The Menstrual Cycle and Other Parameters Affecting Breast Disease and Detection

Linda L. Coughlin

INTRODUCTION

Breast carcinoma is the leading malignancy in American women. One out of eleven women will develop breast cancer in the United States this year, and approximately 40,000 women were expected to die as a result of this disease in 1986 (Wingo, Layde, Lee, Rubin, & Ory, 1987). As awesome as these statistics are, it is the benign breast problems and their diagnosis and management that plague health care providers and women themselves.

Current research shows that 20–50% of women exhibit signs of fibrocystic breast disease (FBD) during their reproductive years. The most frequent symptoms are palpable masses associated with pain, tenderness, and fullness that generally fluctuate with the menstrual cycle. Although the exact relationship between FBD and cancer is unknown, most practitioners agree that there is an increased risk of developing breast cancer for women with fibrocystic changes, and that these women need close follow-up (Ayers & Gidwani, 1983; Brady et al., 1982; Davis, 1983; Hutchinson et al., 1980; Lundy, 1983; Marchant, Small, & Pinotti, 1983).

Newsome and McLelland (1986) recently warned against relying totally on mammography in the presence of other findings because of its variable false-negative rate, ranging from 5 to 69% in selected studies. Although mammography is the only proved method for detecting nonpalpable breast cancers, 20% of the 4,443 cancers diagnosed in the Breast Center Detection Demonstration Project (BCDDP) were missed using a combination of x-ray mammography and physical examination (Baker, 1982). The University of Michigan site for this 5-year project (UM-BCDDP) screened women with film mammography and physical examination with comparable results (Schmitt & Threatt, 1984).

These studies imply that mammography and physical examination are not sensitive enough for detecting breast cancers in all age groups and indicate the need to investigate and improve on other diagnostic tools to aid in the early detection of breast carcinoma and in defining benign diseases.

A project was undertaken at the Breast Diagnostic Center in Colorado Springs, Colorado, from June to December 1983 to determine what correlations exist between thermography and other evaluation techniques, and in addition, whether there is a relationship between abnormalities identified using these techniques and other parameters. The researcher administered a questionnaire to clients to gather information on menstrual, reproductive, and medical history, and dietary intake (see chapter appendix). The diet information was based on recall of current eating habits. Each client underwent bilateral thermography and physical examination by the author. Several subjects were given additional screening, if ordered, indicated, or desired.

The use of thermography in the diagnosis of breast disease has been controversial since its inception in 1956. Heat, or a rise in body temperature, has frequently been associated with disease, and in past years, an elevated temperature or warm forehead was considered to be a main signal to physicians of a disease process. Love (cited in Milbrath, 1982) hypothesizes that the increased supply of blood to a tumor, rather than the tumor itself, will result in a variation of local skin temperature. It is reasonable to expect that almost any active disease process, benign or malignant, may cause a variation in skin temperature.

Thermography is based on the fact that all tissues emit infrared radiation, electromagnetic waves with wavelengths from 0.75 μm to 1 mm. The infrared spectrum emitted by the human body peaks at 9.3 μm. Since infrared radiation is invisible, special instruments are utilized to detect it. The Breast Diagnostic Center used a contact thermography system from Vectra (Vectra International Corporation, Columbia, Maryland). In contact thermography a sheet of plastic containing heat-sensitive, encapsulated liquid crystals of cholesterol esters is placed against the breast. Infrared radiation causes the cholesterol crystals to change colors, which vary with the energies emitted from the breast surface. The color image on the plate is then photographed while the plate is in contact with the breast. Contact thermography is also known as liquid-crystal thermography (LCT) (Milbrath, 1982).

METHODS

Thermography begins with the client disrobing from the waist up and sitting in a cool room (70–75 °F) with her arms elevated and her hands on the top of her head, or behind her neck, to allow the body temperature to cool. As an alternative, the client may lie on a table with her hands behind her head. All clients were cooled for a minimum of 10 minutes during which time the questionnaire was administered. Thermography was performed during the morning hours, 7:30 a.m. to noon, to reduce the effect of the rising air temperature. Clients were asked to abstain from alcohol for 24 h, smoking for 3 h, and to avoid the use of deodorants, body lotions, perfumes, and makeup on their upper torso. Before thermographs were taken, a sketch was made of the veins and scars on the breasts. Clients were given a rating from T1 to T5 for each breast based on four pictures—a frontal and lateral view of each breast. Ratings were based on a subjective comparison of breast symmetry relative to vascular patterns and areas of increased temperature (Richardson, Cigtay, Grant, & Wang, 1984).

Individuals displaying overt heat discrepancies between breasts, and all lactating women, underwent a "stress test," and the photographs were repeated. The stress test involved placing both hands in a tub of ice water for 45 sec to further cool the breasts and remove potential heat artifacts.

The clients then underwent a complete breast examination. Supra- and subclavicular and axillary lymph nodes were palpated for adenopathy. The breasts were inspected for symmetry, nipple position, dimpling, puckering, vein pattern, size discrepancies, and other abnormalities in three positions: sitting with arms relaxed, raised, and flexed on the hips. The nipples were then checked for discharge, and the breast tissue was compressed for masses. The client was repositioned, lying on her back, with her arms flexed behind her head and both breasts were examined in this position. Any palpable masses were felt by the client, and self-breast examination (SBE) was explained and encouraged to be repeated monthly, after the menses for menstruating women, and at a regular time for postmenopausal or posthysterectomized women.

If additional testing was indicated or ordered, the Center used an Ausonic (Ausonics, New Berlin, Wisconsin) water bath ultrasound and film screen mammography (L Cent, Inc., Boston, Massachusetts). The thermograms, mammograms, and ultrasounds were interpreted by Thomas Ravin, M.D. Biopsies and surgical procedures were performed by private physicians outside the Breast Center.

In March 1987 (4 years after initial evaluation), the author attempted to update the study by telephone contact with the 100 women initially found to be negative for cancer. This new data was analyzed, not on testing procedures, but based on diagnosis of breast cancer versus no change.

RESULTS

The initial study concentrated on correlations between variables and testing procedures. The groups and their frequencies are shown in Table 16-1. The variables investigated are shown in Table 16-2. The sample size of individual diagnoses was so small it was decided to evaluate the data based on two groups, normal and all others, using the Student's *t*-test.

Of the women initially found to be negative for breast cancer (61 women), 61% were contacted in the study update. Twenty-seven women had undergone further mammograms without change; 27 women had experienced no worsening of symptoms and no further testing; 7 women had had biopsies, 2 of which were malignant. The data were analyzed using the SPSSX program comparing two groups—no change after 3½ years (59 women) versus the total number of breast cancers found (4 women). These results, combined with the initial study results, are shown in Table 16-3.

Table 16-1   Groups by Evaluation Technique and Frequencies

Technique	Number	Classification
Examination I	47	Normal
Examination II	55	Masses
		Cystic
		Masses and cystic
Thermogram I	81	Low risks, Th1 Th2
Thermogram II	21	High risks, Th3 Th4 Th5
Mammogram I	24	Normal
Mammogram II	23	P1, Minimal ductal prominence
		P2, Severe ductal prominence
		DY, Severe dysplasia
Ultrasound I	8	Normal
Ultrasound II	39	Fibrous only
		Fibroadenoma
		Fibrous bands and small cysts
		Fibrous bands and large cysts
		Multiple large cysts
		Ductal ectasia
		Fibroadenoma & ductal ectasia
		Fibroadenoma, fibrous bands, small and large cysts
		Ductal ectasia, fibrous bands, small and large cysts
Biopsy I	5	Benign
Biopsy II	2	Malignant

Table 16-2   Variables Investigated for Correlation Between Evaluation Techniques

History	Foods
[a]Age	Total animal
Height	Animal
[a]Weight	Meat
Obesity factor	Bacon
[a]Days from last period	[a]Liver
Age at menarche	[a]Fat
Gravida	[a]Butter
[a]Parity	Fried foods
Abortions	Oil
[a]Number of miscarriages	Nuts
Age of menopause	Dairy
[a]Number of mammograms	Milk
Difficult menopause	[a]Yogurt
Age of hysterectomy	Ice cream
[a]Age of oophorectomy	Cottage cheese
Premeno hormones	Cheese
Postmeno hormones	Poultry
Packs cigarettes	Fish
Years not smoked	Eggs
Economic level	[a]Total methylxanthine
Vitamin B	Colas
Vitamin E	Tea
Thyroid medication	[a]Chocolate
Birth control pills	Cocoa
Hormone replacement	[a]Coffee
Exercise level	[a]White bread
[a]Bowel movements	Whole wheat bread
Wet earwax	Yellow vegetables
Age of first birth	[a]Green vegetables
Breast feeding	Pasta
Bottle feeding	Fruit
[a]Years menstruating	Grain
	Alcohol

[a]Implies significance ($p < .05$).

DISCUSSION

Many factors have been studied for their relationship to breast cancer in an attempt to identify high-risk women, to develop a management program for health care providers, and to provide clues to lifestyle changes that might reduce the incidence of breast cancer. The author defines a risk factor as an attribute that has a positive correlation with the incidence of the disease in question. Table 16-4 lists common risk factors associated with breast disease.

Table 16-3   Significant Parameters by Technique

Variable (no.)	Examination I (47)	Examination II (55)	Thermogram I (81)	Thermogram II (21)	Mammogram I (24)	Mammogram II (23)	Ultrasound I (8)	Ultrasound II (39)	Biopsy I (5)	Biopsy II (2)	Follow-up I (59)	Follow-up II (4)
Age	.001											
Weight	.036											.044
Days from last period		.022										
Parity							.025					
No. of mammograms												.000
No. of miscarriages												.000
Age of oophorectomy												.035
Bowel movements												.000
Years menstruating											.046	
Chocolate		.047										
Fat				.011	.047							
Butter				.006								
Green vegetables									.008			
Coffee												.003
Total methylxanthines												.020
Liver												.001
Yogurt											.002	
White bread											.000	

Numbers represent significant values $p < .05$ by Student's t-test between group 1 (normal) versus group 2 (deviant from normal) for each evaluation modality. The p value is positioned under the group with the increased numerical value for the variable.

Table 16-4 Breast Cancer Risk Factors

Sex	99% women
Age	85% over 45, 67% over 50
Family history	2–9×
Race	5× Caucasians vs. Orientals
	3× Caucasians vs. Blacks
Obesity	2×
Nulliparous	3×
First child after age 30	4×
First child before age 18	1/4×
Early menarche, menses >30 years	1.3×
Menopause after age 50	1.5×
Oophorectomy before age 37	1/3×
Affluent	2×
History of benign breast disease	2–3×
Wet earwax	2×
2 or less bowel movements/week	4×
Endometrial cancer	1.3×
High dietary fats	3×
Conflicting data	
Oral contraceptives	Estrogen replacement therapy
Radiation exposure	Hypothyroidism
Alcohol	Methylxanthine
Breast feeding	Vitamin B complex

Data from Miller and Bulbrook, 1980; Leis, 1980; Petrakis and King, 1981.

Physical examination seemed to be the most consistent predictor of fibrocystic breast disease (FBD) characteristics. Significantly more normal physical examinations were found in older women ($p = .001$), reflecting the tendency of FBD in younger women. Those with abnormal physical examinations, and cancer in the follow-up study, weighed more ($p = .036$, $p = .044$) and were further from the start of their last menstrual period ($p = .022$).

Although no testing procedure correlated with total methylxanthines (coffee, cocoa, tea, chocolate, and cola), significant chocolate consumption ($p = .042$) was found in women with abnormal physical examinations. Methylxanthines have been linked to fibrocystic breast disease (Minton, Foecking, Webster, & Matthews, 1979a). It had been hoped to show a correlation between intake and diagnosis, as caffeine withdrawal has proven to effectively reduce or eliminate the symptoms associated with fibrocystic breast disease (Gonzales, 1980; Minton, Foecking, Webster, & Matthews, 1979b). In the final analysis, women with cancer had consumed significantly more coffee (43 versus 8 cups per week, $p = .003$) and total methylxanthine ($p = .020$).

The published data (Correa, 1981; Committee on Diet, Nutrition, and Cancer, 1982; Enstrom, 1982; Graham et al., 1982; Hems, 1979, 1980; Kinlen, 1982; Kolonel, Hankin, Nomura, & Chu, 1981; Simone, 1983; Wynder, 1980;

Yonemoto, 1980) is conflicting as to the role of nutrition/diet in the development of breast disease. However, it is generally believed that high dietary fat consumption plays a significant part. Although the significance of total fat ($p = .047$) for normal mammograms was higher, it is probably explained by the small sizes of the subgroups and the inability to view each diagnosis as separate. The group with high-risk thermograms reflected a significant increase in butter ($p = .006$) and total fat ($p = .011$) and reinforce the use of thermography as a predictor, rather than a diagnostic, of women who are at risk of developing breast cancer in the future. Gautherie and Gros (1980) found that over one third of women with high-risk thermograms developed histologically confirmed cancers within 5 years.

The only significant dietary factor protecting women from biopsy-proved cancer versus women with benign biopsies was green vegetables ($p = .008$). However, when comparing the total number of women with breast cancer (4) versus the no-change group (59), women with cancer ate significantly more liver ($p = .001$) and less white bread ($p = .000$) and yogurt ($p = .002$). They also had significantly more bowel movements per week ($p = .008$), which contradicts the current literature (Petrakis & King, 1981).

Several menstrual and reproductive factors are thought to influence breast cancer. According to studies (Leis, 1980; Miller & Bulbrook, 1980), prolonged menstrual activity associated with early menarche and later menopause increases the risk for developing breast cancer. This association was not proved in the initial study even when correcting for number of births. However, the follow-up analysis found that the women with cancer had significant ($p = .046$) shorter periods of menstrual activity (32 versus 36 years). When this factor was corrected for births, the significance was not found.

Table 16-5   Comparison of Risk Factors for Women with Breast Cancer

Risk factor client	Women diagnosed with breast cancer			
	1	2	3	4
Age	39	62	51	46
Family history of breast cancer	Paternal great aunt	Sister	Mother, sister Paternal aunt	Maternal great aunt
Obesity	0–19% over	20% over	0–19% over	Desired weight
Age at first term pregnancy	19	23	44	46
Age at menarche	13	15	14	11
Age of menopause	N.A.	47	44	46
History of benign breast problems	No	Yes Biopsy	Biopsy ×3	Pain
Breast or bottle fed	Breast	Bottle	Bottle	Bottle

Table 16-6   Comparison of Evaluation Techniques for Women with Breast Cancer

| Evaluation technique client | Women diagnosed with breast cancer | | | |
	1	2	3	4
Cancerous breast	Left	Right	Right	Right
Examination	Left mass	Thickening right	Normal	Right & left masses
Thermogram	Normal	Abnormal left	Abnormal left	Normal
Mammogram	FBD	Not Done	Severe ductal prominence	Not done
Ultrasound	FBD, left & right	Fibroadenoma, right	Fibroadenoma, left	Solid cyst, right

Parity (age at first birth) and oophorectomy before age 37 are thought to be protective against breast cancer (Leis, 1980; Miller & Bulbrook, 1980). Those women with normal ultrasounds had significantly more births ($p = .025$).

The follow-up analysis found that the women with cancer were significantly older at oophorectomy (44 versus 36 years, $p = .035$), thus supporting the protective effect theory for early removal of ovaries. Age at first birth did not correlate in any analysis, but the women with cancer had significantly more miscarriages (3 versus 1.28) ($p = .000$).

The influence of estrogen replacement therapy (Gambrell, 1982; Hammond, Maxson, & Wayne, 1982; Nachtigall, Nachtigall, & Beckman, 1979; Wingo et al., 1987) for postoophorectomized or postmenopausal women continues to be debated. Although it was not significant ($p = .081$), women with cancer used less postmenopausal hormones (10 versus 81 months).

Recent studies (Miller et al., 1986) are indicating no increased risk of developing breast cancer in prior oral contraceptive users. This study did not show any correlation with prior oral contraceptive use. Some authors (Petrakis & King, 1981) have proposed that thyroid medication may also offer protection against breast cancer. This was not proven by this study.

A comparison of the four clients with biopsy-proved malignancies (Table 16-5) revealed few common risk factors and even contradictions of others. Table 16-6 compares the evaluation techniques and their inconsistencies, perhaps a reflection of the fact that the sample size is small and that breast cancer remains a complicated disease to diagnose.

CONCLUSION

There was no consistent predictor of breast cancer and correlation between the testing methods used in the study. Therefore, a multidisciplinary approach, respecting the advantages and disadvantages of the different diagnostic techniques, is recommended when evaluating women seeking diagnosis and treatment of breast masses, pain, or other complaints.

However, the data imply that more normal values for some tests may be found in the follicular phase of the menstrual cycle and after some dietary and lifestyle modifications. These findings may allow practitioners to better educate their clients as to the best time for breast self-examination and scheduling of screening procedures and as to dietary changes that may be associated with reducing their symptoms and, perhaps, risk for developing breast disease.

REFERENCES

Ayers, J. W. T., & Gidwani, G. P. (1983). The "luteal breast": Hormonal and sonographic investigation of benign breast disease in patients with cystic mastalgia. *Fertility and Sterility, 40*(6), 779–784.

Baker, L. (1982). Breast cancer detection demonstration project: Five-year summary report. *A Cancer Journal for Clinicians, 32*(4), 194–225.

Brady, L. J., McBride, C. M., Moore, A., Shirley, R. L., Smith, F., & Jankowski, N. W. (1982). Assessing the risk for breast cancer. *Patient Care, 16*(5), 21–43.

Committee on Diet, Nutrition, and Cancer (1982). *Diet, nutrition and cancer.* Washington, DC: National Academy Press.

Correa, P. (1981). Epidemiological correlation between diet and cancer frequency. *Cancer Research, 41*(9), 3685–3690.

Davis, S. R. (1983). The breast lumps that aren't cancer. *RN, 46*(8), 30–33.

Enstrom, J. E. (1982). Assessing human epidemiologic data on diet as an etiologic factor in cancer development. *Bulletin of the New York Academy of Medicine, 58*(3), 313–322.

Gambrell, R. D. (1982). The menopause: Benefits and risks of estrogen-progestogen replacement therapy. *Fertility and Sterility, 37*(4), 457–474.

Gautherie, M., & Gros, C. M. (1980). Breast thermography and cancer risk prediction. *Cancer, 45,* 51–56.

Gonzales, E. R. (1980). For others, methylxanthine withdrawal may work. Medical News, *Journal of the American Medical Association, 244*(10), 1078–1079.

Graham, S., Marshall, J., Mettlin, C., Rzepka, T., Nemoto, T., & Byers, T. (1982). Diet in the epidemiology of breast cancer. *American Journal of Epidemiology, 116*(1), 68–77.

Hammond, C. B., & Maxson, W. S. (1982). Current status of estrogen replacement therapy for the menopause. *Fertility and Sterility, 37*(1), 5–25.

Hems, G. (1979). Associations between breast cancer mortality rates, child-bearing and diet in the United Kingdom. *British Journal of Cancer, 41,* 429–437.

Hems, G. (1980). Epidemiological characteristics of breast cancer in middle and late age. *British Journal of Cancer, 24,* 226–234.

Hutchinson, W. B., Thomas, D. B., Hamlin, W. B., Roth, G. J., Peterson, A. V., and Williams, B. (1980). Risk of breast cancer in women with benign breast disease. *Journal of the National Cancer Institute,* 13–20.

Kinlen, L. J. (1982, April 24). Meat and fat consumption and cancer mortality: A study of strict religious orders in Britain. *Lancet, i,* 946–949.

Kolonel, L. N., Hankin, J. H., Nomura, A. M., & Chu, S. Y. (1981). Dietary fat intake and cancer incidence among five ethnic groups in Hawaii. *Cancer Research, 41*(9), 3727–3728.

Leis, H. P. (1980). Risk factors for breast cancer: An update. *Breasts: Diseases of the Breast, 6*(4), 21–26.

Lundy, J. (1983). Lumps: When is close follow-up appropriate? *Contemporary OB/ GYN,* 196–209.

Marchant, D., Small, E. C., & Pinotti, J. A. (1983). The breast: Management. *The Female Patient, 8,* 19–29.

Milbrath, J. R. (1982). Thermography. In L. Bassett & R. H. Gold, *Mammography, thermography and ultrasound in breast cancer detection* (pp. 143–149). New York: Grune & Stratton.

Miller, A. B., & Bulbrook, R. D. (1980). The epidemiology and etiology of breast cancer. *The New England Journal of Medicine, 303*(21), 1246–1248.

Miller, D. R., Rosenberg, L., Kaufman, D. W., Schottenfeld, D., Stolley, P. D., & Shapiro, S. (1986). Breast cancer risk in relation to early oral contraceptive use. *Obstetrics and Gynecology, 68*(6), 863–868.

Minton, J. P., Foecking, M. K., Webster, D. J. T., & Matthews, R. H. (1979a). Caffeine, cyclic nucleotides and breast disease. *Surgery, 86*(1), 105–108.

Minton, J. P., Foecking, M. K., Webster, D. J. T., & Matthews, R. H. (1979b). Response to fibrocystic disease to caffeine withdrawal and correlation of cyclic nucleotides with breast disease. *American Journal of Obstetrics Gynecology, 244*(10), 157–158.

Nachtigall, L. E., Nachtigall, R. H., Nachtigall, R. D., & Beckman, E. M. (1979). Estrogen replacement therapy, II: A prospective study in the relationship to carcinoma and cardiovascular and metabolic problems. *Obstetrics and Gynecology, 54*(1), 74–79.

Newsome, J. F., & McLelland, R. (1986). A word of caution concerning mammography. *Journal of the American Medical Association, 255*(4), 528.

Petrakis, N. L., & King, E. B. (1981, November 28). Cytological abnormalities in nipple aspirates of breast fluid from women with severe constipation. *Lancet, ii,* 1203–1204.

Richardson, J. D., Cigtay, O. S., Grant, E. G., & Wang, P. C. (1984). Imaging of the breast. *Medical Clinics of North America, 68*(6), 1481–1514.

Schmitt, E. L., & Threatt, B. (1984). Characteristics of breast cancer in an incident cancer population. *American Journal of Radiology, 143,* 403–406.

Simone, C. B. (1983). *Cancer and nutrition.* New York: McGraw-Hill.

Wingo, P. A., Layde, P. M., Lee, N. C., Rubin, G., & Ory, H. W. (1987). The risk of breast cancer in post menopausal women who have used estrogen replacement therapy. *Journal of the American Medical Association, 275*(2), 209–215.

Wynder, E. L. (1980). Dietary factors related to breast cancer. *Cancer,* 899–904.

Yonemoto, R. H. (1980). Breast cancer in Japan and the United States. *Archives of Surgery, 115*(9–80), 1056–1062.

APPENDIX

Questionnaire

Name _____ Phone _____

Age _____ Date of birth _____ SSN _____

Height _____ Weight _____ LMP _____

Age of menarche _____ Gravida _____ Parity _____ Abortion _____

Age of menopause ____ Difficult ____ Hysterectomy ____ Oophorectomy ____

Hormones (what, when, for how long) _____

Pregnancy   1   2   3   4   5   6   7   8   9   10   11

    Age

    Outcome

    Feeding

Yearly income _____

Smoking: Number _____ Packs/day _____ Yrs _____ Yrs quit _____

Current medication _____

Current vitamins _____

Family history breast problems   Mat _____ Pat _____

Personal history breast problems _____

Do you feel your breasts mimic the maternal or paternal side? _____

Exercise each week _____

Bowel movements per week _____ Earwax wet/dry   Amount _____

Average number of servings weekly:

3 oz meat (beef, pork) _____   3 oz poultry _____

3 oz fish, seafood _____   3 oz liver _____

3 oz bacon, bologna, hot dogs, processed or smoked meat _____

Slices white bread _____   Slices whole grain bread _____

Butter, pats, tsp _____   Oil, salad dressing,
                             mayo, 1 tbsp _____

Fried foods, no. times _____   Coffee, cups _____

Tea, cups _____   Colas, 12 oz _____

Chocolate, oz _____   Cocoa, cups _____

Alcohol: liquor, 1 oz; beer, 12 oz; wine, 4 oz _____

Sweets _____   Eggs _____

Milk, 4 oz _____   Yogurt, 4 oz _____

Cottage cheese, ricotta, 4 oz _____   Ice cream, 4 oz _____

Cheese, 1 oz _____   Nuts, 1 oz _____

Green vegetables, 1/2 cup _____   Yellow vegetables, 1/2 cup _____

Fruit: 1/2 cup, one serving _____   Pasta, potatoes, 1/2 cup _____

Grains, beans, rice, dry peas, 1/2 cup _____

Number of chest x-rays _____

Number of mammograms _____

Part Three

Menopause:
Normative Transition
or Illness Event?

Menopause, a universal event in women's lives, is experienced by women in a variety of ways. These chapters contribute to an understanding of women's menopausal experiences and methods for studying them. Guice (Chapter 17) examined two explanations for initiation of the menopausal hot flash by contrasting a pathological orientation with a physiological orientation. The evidence she examined supports the concept of the hot flash as a thermoregulatory adaptive mechanism.

McElmurry and Huddleston (Chapter 18) viewed menopausal experiences through analysis of women's stories. They found that perimenopausal women's self-care responses could be understood when examined in relation to their life perspectives, health experiences, health explanations, and health relationships.

Bareford (Chapter 19) examined the relationship of attitudes toward menopause, recent life changes, coping method, and menopausal symptoms. Her results support the importance of negative attitudes toward menopause and recent life changes in women's symptom experiences. In her study, positive attitudes toward menopause seemed to ameliorate the negative effects of recent life changes on symptoms.

Glazer and Rozman (Chapter 20) considered the concepts of marital adjustment, life stress, attitudes toward menopause, and menopausal symptoms and their measurement. Their critical appraisal of commonly used instruments raises cautions for menstrual cycle researchers.

Chapter 17

Assumptions Underlying Two Hypotheses of Hot Flash Initiation and Evidence Pertaining to Their Validity

Elizabeth E. Guice

INTRODUCTION

Reduction in levels of circulating estrogens has been accepted as the underlying condition that results in the menopausal hot flash. However, the exact mechanism(s) by which the withdrawal of estrogen acts to produce a flash is not known. In the United States, the prevailing hypothesis has tended to direct research toward hormonal or biochemical products that affect the hypothalamic thermoregulatory center—physiological monitoring of the flashes having become more or less relegated to providing indicators of the presence of a flash. In the United Kingdom and Europe, more emphasis has been placed on circulatory variables (Coope, Williams, & Patterson, 1978; Sturdee, Wilson, Pipili, & Crocker, 1978; Ginsburg, Swinhoe, & O'Reilly, 1981; Ginsburg, Hardiman, & O'Reilly, 1989; Nesheim & Saetre, 1982; Duncan, 1982; Brincat, Detrafford, Lafferty, & Studd, 1984; Rees & Barlow, 1988).

In addition, although the flash is generally accepted as thermoregulatory (Tataryn et al., 1980; Kronenberg & Downey, 1987), simultaneous study of both *heat production* and *heat elimination* in hot flashing women has not been reported. Since heat loss is primarily effected by removal of heat brought to the skin surface by the circulatory system (with or without sweating), circulatory changes resulting from estrogen withdrawal could be expected to affect heat loss capability.

Thus, two almost diametrically opposed hypotheses of immediate hot flash causation can be presented, with opposed implications for any treatment other than hormonal replacement therapy (HRT). Most of the experimental data and subjective report is not under dispute but is commonly accepted. The exception in unpublished data, in part presented here, on variables not reported by other researchers. There is no basic disagreement on the physiological pattern of the hot flash. It is in the interpretation of data held in common that the two hypotheses differ.

The two hypotheses diverge most importantly in regard to the assumed normality or pathology of the hot flash episode. The hypotheses will be presented, including their experimental bases. The assumptions underlying each hypothesis will explicitly be stated, together with experimental evidence in support or opposition to the extent that such evidence exists.

HYPOTHESES

Hypothesis 1

Hypothesis 1 (H1) of an altered setpoint is the current consensual one (Tataryn et al., 1980). It states that the flash results from the pulsatile release of some unknown biochemical, which causes a transient lowering of the setpoint located in the thermoregulatory center of the hypothalamus, thus initiating activity to effect an immediate loss of heat to make core temperature conform to the new, pathologically low setpoint; as this chemical gradually dissipates, the setpoint gradually returns to normal and core temperature rises accordingly.

Experimental Basis

Hypothesis 1 was developed to conform to what was later found to be a faulty premise, that a pulsatile release of luteinizing hormone (LH) preceded the flash and that it was this hormone that lowered the setpoint (Meldrum et al., 1979). When further study demonstrated that this interpretation was untenable (Lightman, Jacobs, & Maguire, 1982), the hypothesis was retained by postulating the existence of some other biochemical, as yet undiscovered (Kronenberg & Downey, 1987). No suggestion has been offered to account for the pulsatile release of such a chemical, nor is any suggestion offered to account for the known relationship of ambient temperature (Coope et al., 1978; Molnar, 1980) and other heat sources (Voda, 1981) to number and/or severity of the flashes.

Hypothesis 2

Hypothesis 2 (H2) of diminished heat loss has been offered by the author. It proposes that one result of altered levels of circulating female steroids is to reduce peripheral or specifically cutaneous circulation and sweating with a resulting reduction of normal heat loss capability; then, under the usual conditions of temperature and humidity, heat will build up within the body core and require intermittent release through "emergency" and probably sympathetic nervous system (SNS) initiated action—a coarse, rather than fine tuning—involving an active shunting of blood to the cutaneous blood vessels. The activities involved in the shunting of blood from the core to the body surface represent the flash as objectively monitored and subjectively experienced. Prodromata experienced by some women would be assumed to result from an awareness of the internal changes of impending or impeded attempts to make the shunt.

Experimental Basis

Over a series of exploratory monitoring sessions using a variety of sensors and sensor placements, the tentative hypothesis was formed that a gradual rise in core temperature (whether oral, tympanic, or esophageal), unaccompanied by sporadic increases in finger pulse volume (FPV, measured by photoelectric plethysmography and indicating increased blood flow in the finger tips), would be followed by a hot flash. The tracing of FPV for some subjects almost flattened out between flashes. This suggested inhibition of heat loss activity, which was borne out by consistent self-report that external or internal heat increased the number and/or severity of the flashes.

One hot flash subject was monitored by thermography throughout a flash. The pattern of increase in surface heat during a flash was identical to that described by Eberhart and Trezek (1973) in an account of rewarming after hypothermic surgery, although that account used temperature of the big toe and thermography of the foot and lower leg where Guice and Hoekstra (in preparation) monitored the chest, neck, hand, and arm. The interpretation given by Eberhart and Trezek was that when internal temperature rose to a sufficient level, blood was shunted to the peripheral system, appearing first in the digits where arteriovenous shunts speeded its arrival, then gradually reaching the capillaries where such shunts were not available.

METHODS

Guice and Wirth (in preparation) then conducted a study designed to examine both heat production and heat loss, reasoning that either heat production was intermittently increased or heat elimination was faulty. Eleven postmenopausal volunteers, six with and four without hot flashes, were subjects for the study.

The eleventh was tested twice, once unmedicated and experiencing severe hot flashes, and again under HRT and being symptom free. Recording sessions lasted long enough for two flashes and the interflash interval in hot flash subjects and for an equal duration for control subjects. Heat production was monitored by measurement of oxygen utilization per minute. The rectal site for monitoring core temperature was used, since esophageal and tympanic sites were blocked by the presence of equipment for the measurement of oxygen use. Heat loss was monitored at three sites. Digital sweating (skin conductance digital, SCd) was chosen as an indicator of sympathetic nervous system arousal and also, following Allen, Robinson, and Roddie (1978) and Wilcott (1963), as an indicator of thermoregulatory sweating. Forearm sweating (skin conductance forearm, SCfa) at the volar site was chosen as an indicator of parasympathetic activity (Wenger, 1948) and also as an indicator of sweating at this acknowledged thermoregulatory sweating site. FPV by photoelectric plethysmography was chosen as a direct indicator of increased blood flow in the skin of the palmar surface of the finger tip, a site with arteriovenous anastomoses, and hence providing earlier indication of blood flow increase than change in temperature at the proximal phalanx as used by Meldrum et al. (1979) for an objective index of the occurrence of a hot flash. FPV was recorded in millimeters of pen deflection and converted to millivolts in terms of the gain setting.

RESULTS

The most remarkable finding was that subjects with hot flashes displayed markedly diminished levels of sweating on fingertips and of pulse volume on fingertips in the interflash interval as compared to asymptomatic subjects; these parameters reached levels equivalent to those for control subjects only at the time of the hot flash. In addition, forearm sweating was intermittent throughout the session for controls but occurred only within the flash episode for hot flash subjects (Figures 17-1, 17-2, & 17-3).

No difference was found between groups in oxygen consumption (heat production). No difference was found in amount or rate of decline of rectal temperature to nadir and rise thereafter (Table 17-1). Average individual maximum values for the two sweat variables and the finger circulation variable were *not* significantly different, but average mean and minimum values for the first two variables were significantly lower for the hot flash group (Table 17-2). This, together with the very obvious differences found in the pattern of activity at the three heat-loss sites during the core temperature decline, supports H2.

In hot flash subjects, the synchronous activity at the three monitored sites, identical with the objective indications of a hot flash as previously described in the literature, was accompanied by the subjective experience of a flash. Control subjects, on the other hand, displayed only intermittent and unsynchronized activity at these same three sites throughout the entire recording session.

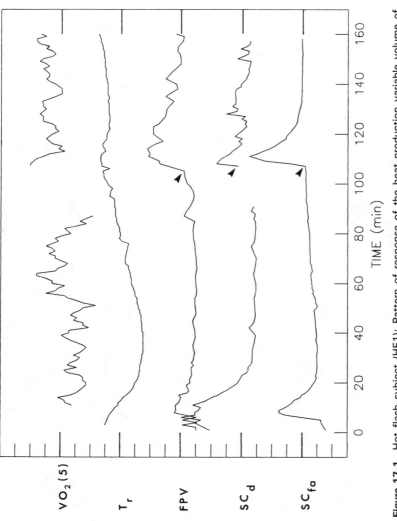

Figure 17-1 Hot flash subject (HF1): Pattern of response of the heat production variable volume of oxygen consumed per minute expressed as a running average over a 5-min interval [$VO_2(5)$], rectal temperature (Tr), and three heat-loss variables (FPV, SCd, and SCfa) over a 160-min recording session. The units are standard deviation values for each variable, computed for this individual. Arrows mark the start of the flash response for that variable. The longer and darker lines on the vertical axis mark the mean value for each variable, and the shorter lines mark the ± standard deviation values associated with those mean values.

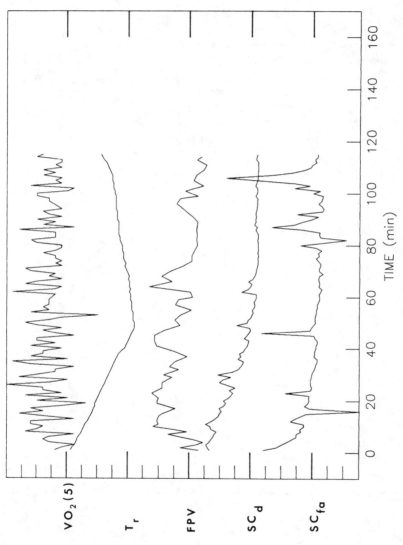

Figure 17-2 Control subject (C1): Pattern of response of the heat production variable volume of oxygen consumed per minute expressed as a running average over a 5-min interval [$VO_2(5)$], rectal temperature (T_r), and three heat-loss variables (FPV, SCd, and SCfa) over a 120-min recording session. The units are standard deviation values for each variable, computed for this individual. The longer and darker lines on the vertical axis mark the mean value for each variable, and the shorter lines mark the ± standard deviation values associated with those mean values.

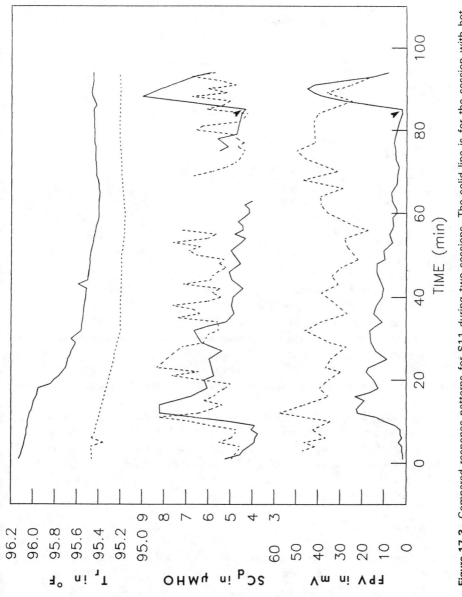

Figure 17-3 Compared response patterns for S11 during two sessions. The solid line is for the session with hot flashes; the dashed line is for the session when she was medicated and flash free. Arrows mark the start of the flash response for that variable.

Table 17-1 Comparisons (t-Test) Between Hot Flash and Control Subjects for Rectal Temperature Parameters

| Variable | Mean | | t (6 DF) |
	C (4 Ss)	HF (4 Ss)	
Decline to nadir			
Temp (degrees F)	0.54	0.60	0.45 NS
Time (min)	43.25	57.0	1.13 NS
Rise after nadir			
Temp (degrees F)	0.42	0.27	0.96 NS
Rate (degrees/min)	0.0060	0.0060	—

Key: C = control subjects, 4 in number; HF = hot flash subjects, also 4 in number; t = t scores with 6 degrees of freedom (DF).

DISCUSSION

Although the change from active to passive state may have caused the initial drop in core temperature as muscular activity (and hence metabolic activity) decreased, this would not account for the difference in synchrony of heat loss activity between the subject groups. The difference suggests impaired heat loss capability between flashes.

Assumptions Underlying the Hypotheses and Existing Evidence

Since hypotheses follow logically from their assumptions and tests of hypotheses follow logically from those hypotheses, and since the application of logic is itself straightforward, a key factor in experimental research must be the testing of such underlying assumptions. This does not appear to have taken place in regard to H1 because they were never made explicit and hence were not available for direct experimental test.

Basic Assumption

The two hypotheses diverge most importantly in regard to the physiological function of the hot flash episode. H1 assumes pathology, implying the flash serves no valid thermoregulatory function. The flash is used as evidence for the existence of and is at the same time declared to be a response to an aberrant chemical that has yet to be found. H2 assumes the flash serves a valid thermo-regulatory function as an adaptation or adjustment to reduced peripheral circu-lation and sweating.

Possibly as a result of the assumption that the hot flash is the pathology and a focus on medical treatment of the symptom, proponents of H1 have directed their attention to the hot flash episode itself and have shown less concern for what goes on between flashes. Physiological indicators have been used primar-ily to objectify the flash and define its start in a clinical rather than investigative mode. Choice of sites for placement of sensors was in terms of utility rather than the physiological meaning of changes at that site (skin temperature and sweating to be discussed later). On the other hand, the author of H2 began by assuming an abnormality in thermoregulation, broadly defined to include both heat production and heat loss. Hence, attention was paid to baseline and

Table 17-2   *t*-Test Comparisons Between Control and Hot Flash Subject Groups

Parameter	Finger pulse volumes (in microvolts)		*t*	DF	Sig
	C(n = 3)	HF(n = 6)			
Minima	12.42	5.92	1.94	7	$p < .05$
Means	32.28	14.38	4.18	7	$p < .005$
Maxima	58.58	39.77	1.27	7	NS

Parameter	Digital skin conductance (in micromhos)		*t*	DF	Sig
	C(n = 3)	HF(n = 5)			
Minima	5.10	2.95	4.14	6	$p < .005$
Means	7.05	4.39	3.38	6	$p < .01$
Maxima	12.25	9.39	0.83	6	NS

Parameter	Forearm skin conductance (in micromhos)		*t*	DF	Sig
	C(n = 3)	HF(n = 5)			
Minima	3.33	3.55	−0.180	6	NS
Means	4.02	4.38	−0.269	6	NS
Maxima	5.55	6.27	−0.393	6	NS

Minimum values for each variable were determined for each subject. These individual minima were averaged for control (C) and hot flash (HF) subject groups. Then the means of the two subject groups were compared by *t*-test (*t*) with appropriate degrees of freedom (DF). The same procedure was followed for individual maximum scores and for mean scores.

changes in a wider range of pertinent variables and recording sites and throughout the entire hot flash cycle.

Subordinate Assumptions

Following from the divergence concerning whether the hot flash or the thermal regulation between flashes is the abnormality, the two hypotheses diverge in how "normal" is defined for three major variables and in the selection of monitoring variables and sensor sites. Changes in those variables during the flash episode, in consequence, are interpreted differently.

Core Temperature   H1 arbitrarily defines the core temperature found just before the beginning of the hot flash as normal. By this definition, the observed decline of temperature during the flash must be abnormal in its presence and, by inference, abnormal in amount.

H2 assumes the temperature just before the flash to be at a level that would normally initiate heat loss activities. By this definition, decline of temperature during the flash would be a step in the right direction, although coarse tuning might involve a more abrupt decline and a possible overshoot. Core temperature would be expected to oscillate more widely than when fine tuning was possible.

Existing Evidence   Useful norms for core temperature cannot be established for lack of sufficient evidence. No norms have been reported in the literature for either males or females of postmenopausal age, and very few postmenopausal women without hot flashes have been tested. In a few instances, the experimental design was intended to compare the same subjects when on HRT and when unmedicated (Brincat et al., 1984; Rees & Barlow, 1988; Mashchak, Kletzky, Artal, & Mishell, 1984), but even then the data has not been analyzed with this exact question in mind.

As for changes during the flash, evidence from Guice (in preparation) is that both hot flash and control subjects showed the same core temperature decline over the same time span (20–30 min) at the start of the sessions. Average rectal temperature for the two groups was the same. This would indicate the hypothalamic thermoregulatory center was successful in maintaining normal core temperature, although by coarse tuning.

Surface Temperature and Circulation   H1 again arbitrarily defines as normal the finger temperature just before a flash (Meldrum et al., 1979), and thus increased surface temperature is also, by definition, abnormal during the flash; the site chosen to monitor skin temperature, the dorsum of the proximal phalanx of the third finger, was chosen for its ease of monitoring (Meldrum et al., 1979), not for its physiological relevance to thermal regulation. Since skin temperature results from blood flow, the implication is that blood flow just before a flash is normal, wherever measured and by whatever means. Consequently, the observed increase in peripheral circulation during the hot flash is, by definition, abnormal.

H2 assumes peripheral, or more precisely, cutaneous circulation to be reduced before the flash, hence predicts an increase during the flash with concomitant rise in surface temperature, and declares the levels of cutaneous circulation and temperature to be more nearly normal during a flash than between flashes.

Existing Evidence   The weight of what evidence is available supports H2. Brincat et al. (1984) and Rees and Barlow (1988) agree that low levels of estrogen result in diminished peripheral, or cutaneous (as they also used the photoelectric plethysmograph that measures blood flow in superficial capillaries of the skin) circulation of the fingertips between flashes, and that HRT reverses the effect to some extent but does not fully restore it to normal levels. Mashchak et al. (1984) also found changes in this direction for both finger temperature and FPV (using photoelectric plethysmography) when the same subjects were tested under both HRT and unmedicated conditions. Tooke, Tindall, & McNicol (1981) found similar differences in circulation within the terminal capillary loops of the finger nailfold during different stages of the menstrual cycle in younger women; this methodology is the "gold standard" for measuring peripheral blood flow, providing absolute values rather than the relative values of other methods. Ginsburg et al. (1989) show differences in levels and changes in circulatory variables monitored in the hand and in the arm; Sessler and Rubenstein (1989) clarify anatomical and thermoregulatory differences between these two sites and offer information on skin-surface temperature gradients and comparisons of core temperature measurement sites.

As to the pathological nature of the circulatory increase, Nesheim and Saetre (1982) report that changes in circulation (measured by forearm pulse velocity) during a hot flash were identical with those found during a sudden increase of ambient temperature. The similarity in thermographic record of rewarming after hypothermic surgery, as reported by Eberhart and Trezek (1973) and of finger, hand, and arm during a hot flash, also testifies to the flash as being a normal circulatory shunt from core to periphery.

Sweat Function as Indicated by Skin Conductance   H1 does not specifically define "normal" sweating levels, but indirectly assumes the level before the flash to be the norm, since skin conductance change on the manubrium is the designated indicator of hot flash start (Erlik et al., 1981) and a criterion for the presence of an objective flash (Silverman, Bajorek, Lomax, & Tataryn, 1981; Tataryn et al., 1980). Reports in the literature are almost totally confined to skin conductance measures on the obvious hot flash areas of sternum, forehead, and cheeks (but for Sturdee et al., 1978, see later discussion).

H2 postulated SNS involvement in emergency heat loss activity and predicts the abrupt rise of digital skin conductance at the start of the hot flash as an indication of such emergency action. Reduced sweating (skin conductance) throughout the interflash interval on the traditional heat loss sites, such as the forearm, would be expected if there is a reduced heat loss capability. Reduced sweating at the digital site between flashes was not predicted, but should have been since that is a site of thermoregulatory sweating, discussed later.

Existing Evidence   No evidence is available in regard to normal skin conductance levels of forehead, cheeks, or manubrium sterni, and normal digital skin conductance has not been defined as such. There are tremendous differences between subjects at the digital sites, and Kuno (1956) has documented great differences in patterns and amounts of heat regulatory sweating in male subjects.

Observed changes in digital skin conductance support the idea that the flash includes SNS arousal (Sturdee et al., 1978; Guice, in preparation). This is also supported by studies of catecholamine changes (reviewed in Kronenberg & Downey, 1987). Thermal sweating has been shown to include palmar and plantar sites (Wilcott, 1963; Allen, Robinson, & Roddie, 1978). This results from the presence of arteriovenous anastomoses, which are also found in the lips, nose, and ears of humans. The Guice and Wirth (in preparation) results show digital skin conductance to be continuously low between flashes in hot flash subjects, lower than the minimum for controls. Cessation of forearm sweating between flashes (Guice & Wirth, in preparation) further supports the heat retention position of H2.

Definition of the Hot Flash   H1 requires a rise in finger temperature (at the third finger dorsum site) of either 0.5 or 1 °C, accompanied by a rapid increase in skin resistance over the manubrium; the rapid change in skin resistance signals the start of the flash best (Tataryn et al., 1980). Subjective awareness is more or less required.

H2 includes all physiological changes that have been found to accompany a flash, when they occur together in the observed sequence, whether or not there is subjective awareness.

Experimental Evidence   Mashchak et al. (1984), Kronenberg, Cote, Linkie, Dyrenfurth, and Downey (1984), and Guice (in preparation) have tabulated the sequence of physiological and subjective symptoms of a flash, which demonstrate that several other measurable events have occurred before the two that were selected by H1 as criteria. These include increased respiratory rate and amplitude, the variables that exhibited the earliest change in Guice's preliminary studies. Early respiratory changes have also been found by Kindlen and Munro (1988). This can be interpreted as representing the thermoregulatory mechanism of hyperventilation, as found in a current reexamination of the data for oxygen, carbon dioxide, and minute volume from the Guice and Wirth study (in preparation).

The arbitrary definition of hot flash start found in H1 is misleading in the extreme. It is too narrow and has tended to restrict the variety of sensors and sensor sites utilized. As one consequence, faulty time relationships with hormonal and sleep variables are declared (Erlik et al., 1981; Gonen, Sharf, & Lavie, 1986).

Furthermore, arbitrary standards of how much rise in temperature must occur before a hot flash is authenticated have served to obscure the evidence that has led several researchers (including Kronenberg & Downey, 1987) to suggest that many women may demonstrate the same symptoms in milder form, below a subjective threshold of awareness, making both the daily incidence and the number of women experiencing the syndrome even greater than is now reported.

CONCLUSION

Although evidence thus far is too scanty to permit a secure choice between hypotheses, what evidence is available supports H2 rather than H1. Furthermore, the assumption of a physiological basis for the flash is more believable than to postulate an unknown chemical acting on a hypothetical setpoint. Indeed, even the existence of a firm setpoint for core temperature is not supported by evidence presented in hot flash literature, where the exact core temperature immediately preceding a flash is shown to vary (see figures in Molnar, 1975, 1979). There are other theories than setpoint ones to account for thermal regulation (Houdas & Ring, 1982).

Additionally, the setpoint hypothesis offers no rationale for the observed relationship between hot flash occurrence and thermal events. The heat retention hypothesis, H2, is consistent with the many reports of the relationship of hot flash number and severity to ambient temperature and humidity, to activity and tension level, to ingestion of alcohol and hot drinks, to reduced convection as when under covers at night, to nearness to hot stoves or ovens, and so on. Germaine and Freedman (1984) ensured that their subjects produced a flash by the application of heat to the abdomen. Kronenberg and Barnard (1990) have controlled ambient temperature and showed that number and severity of flashes increase when ambient temperature is increased. Women with hot flashes consider themselves to have a heat loss problem, and they respond by reducing household temperature when possible and dressing in natural fibers and loose, layered clothing that permits greater heat loss (Voda, 1981).

It is hoped that further research will be guided by the explicit statement of what have been implicit assumptions. The assumption of H1 that the hot flash represents pathology would make almost all postmenopausal women abnormal in this regard, for no physiological purpose. Until actual norms have been established for core temperature and cutaneous circulation, it would be a mistake to continue to define preflash values as normal. It is also a mistake to continue to confine observations only to those variables already reported in print.

From the standpoint of therapy, there is a need to determine whether the flash itself or reduced peripheral circulation is the abnormality. If it is true that peripheral circulation is reduced, this may have ramifications in other problems of the postmenopausal years, including increase in Reynaud's disease.

REFERENCES

Allen, J. A., Robinson, P. H., & Roddie, I. C. (1978). Thermal sweating from the palms and soles. *Proceedings of the Physiological Society, 35P and 36P.*

Brincat, M., Detrafford, J. C., Lafferty, K., & Studd, J. W. W. (1984). Peripheral vasomotor control and menopausal flushing—A preliminary report. *British Journal of Obstetrics and Gynecology, 91,* 1107–1110.

Coope, J., Williams, S., & Patterson, J. S. (1978). A study of the effectiveness of propanolol in menopausal hot flushes. *British Journal of Obstetrics and Gynecology, 85,* 472–475.

Duncan, S. L. B. (1982). Menopausal flushing: Where now? *British Journal of Obstetrics and Gynecology, 89,* 975–976.

Eberhart, R. C. & Trezek, G. J. (1973). Central and peripheral rewarming patterns in postoperative cardiac patients. *Critical Care Medicine, 1,* 239–251.

Erlik, Y., Tataryn, I. V., Meldrum, D. R., Lomax, P., Bajorek, J., & Judd, H. L. (1981). Association of waking episodes with menopausal hot flushes. *Journal of the American Medical Association, 245*(17), 1741–1744.

Germaine, L. M., & Freedman, R. R. (1984). Behavioral treatment of menopausal hot flashes: Evaluation by objective methods. *Journal of Consulting and Clinical Psychology, 52*(6), 1072–1079.

Ginsburg, J., Swinhoe, J., & O'Reilly, B. (1981). Cardiovascular responses during the menopausal hot flush. *British Journal of Obstetrics and Gynecology, 88,* 925–930.

Ginsberg, J., Hardiman, P., & O'Reilly, B. (1989). Peripheral blood flow in menopausal women who have hot flushes and in those who do not. *British Medical Journal, 298,* 1488–1490.

Gonen, R., Sharf, M., & Lavie, P. (1986). The association between mid-sleep waking episodes and hot flushes in post-menopausal women. *Journal of Psychosomatic Obstetrics and Gynecology, 5,* 113–117.

Houdas, Y. & Ring, E. F. (Eds.). (1982). *Human body temperature: Its measurement and regulation.* New York: Plenum Press.

Kindlen, A. S. & Munro, R. E. C. (1988). Respiratory changes during a menopausal hot flush. *Maturitas, 10,* 65–69.

Kronenberg, F. & Barnard, R. M. (1990). Influence of ambient temperature on frequency and intensity of menopausal hot flashes. In M. Flint, F. Kronenberg, & W. Utian (Eds.), *Multidisciplinary perspectives on menopause.* New York: New York Academy of Sciences.

Kronenberg, F., Cote, L. J., Linkie, D. M., Dyrenfurth, I., & Downey, J. A. (1984). Menopausal hot flashes: Thermoregulatory, cardiovascular, and circulating catecholamine and LH changes. *Maturitas, 6,* 31–43.

Kronenberg, F. & Downey, J. A. (1987). Thermoregulatory physiology of menopausal hot flashes: A review. *Canadian Journal of Physiology and Pharmacology, 65,* 1312–1324.

Kuno, Y. (1956). *Human perspiration.* Springfield, Il: Charles C Thomas.

Lightman, S. L., Jacobs, H. S., & Maguire, A. K. (1982). Down-regulation of gonadotrophin secretion in postmenopausal women by a superactive LHRH analogue: Lack of effect on menopausal flushing. *British Journal of Obstetrics and Gynaecology, 89,* 977–980.

Mashchak, C. A., Kletzky, O. A., Artal, R., & Mishell Jr., D. R. (1984). The relation of physiological changes to subjective symptoms in postmenopausal women with and without hot flushes. *Maturitas, 6,* 301–308.

Meldrum, D. R., Shamonki, I. M., Frumar, A. M., Tataryn, I. V., Chang, R. J., & Judd, H. L. (1979). Elevations in skin temperature of the finger as an objective index of postmenopausal hot flashes: Standardization of the technique. *American Journal of Obstetrics and Gynecology, 135,* 713–717.

Molnar, G. W. (1975). Body temperatures during menopausal hot flashes. *Journal of Applied Physiology, 38*(3), 499–503.

Molnar, G. W. (1979). Investigation of hot flashes by ambulatory monitoring. *American Journal of Physiology: Regulatory Integrative Comparative Physiology 6*(3), R306–R310.

Molnar, G. W. (1980). Menopausal hot flashes: Their cycles and relation to air temperature. *Obstetrics and Gynecology, 57,* 52S–55S.

Nesheim, B.-I. & Saetre, T. (1982). Changes in skin blood flow and body temperatures during climacteric hot flushes. *Maturitas, 4,* 49–55.

Rees, M. C., & Barlow, D. H. (1988). Absence of sustained reflex vasoconstriction in women with menopausal flushes. *Human Reproduction, 7,* 823–825.

Sessler, D. I. & Rubenstein, E. H. (1989). In reply. In Correspondence, *Anesthesiology, 70,* 371–372.

Silverman, R. W., Bajorek, J. G., Lomax, P., & Tataryn, I. V. (1981). Monitoring the pathophysiological correlates of postmenopausal hot flushes. *Maturitas, 3,* 39–46.

Sturdee, W., Wilson, K. A., Pipili, E., & Crocker, A. D. (1978). Physiological aspects of menopausal hot flush. *British Medical Journal, 2,* 79–80.

Tataryn, I. V., Lomax, P., Bajorek, J. G., Chesarek, W., Meldrum, D. W., & Judd, H. L. (1980). Postmenopausal hot flushes: A disorder of thermoregulation. *Maturitas, 2,* 101–107.

Tooke, J. E., Tindall, H., & McNicol, G. P. (1981). The influence of a combined oral contraceptive pill and menstrual cycle phase on digital microvascular haemodynamics. *Clinical Sciences, 61*(1), 91–95.

Voda, A. M. (1981). The climacteric hot flash. *Maturitas, 3,* 73–90.

Wenger, M. A. (1948). Studies of autonomic balance in Army Air Force personnel. *Comparative Psychology Monographs, 2,* 173–186.

Wilcott, R. V. (1963). Effects of high environmental temperature in sweating and skin resistance. *Journal of Comparative Physiology and Psychology, 56,* 778–782.

Chapter 18

Perimenopausal Women: Using Women's Stories as a Theoretical Underpinning for Women's Health

Beverly J. McElmurry and Donna S. Huddleston

INTRODUCTION

The authors conducted the study reported here from a women's health perspective that stresses the importance of the lived experience (McBride & McBride, 1981) as a theoretical underpinning for all research with women.

In keeping with Allan and Hall's (1988) challenge to use models other than the medical model when conducting research, we relied on stories from women about their perimenopausal experiences. We agree with Voda and Eliasson (1983), who pioneered efforts to correct the view that menopause is a disease. Rather, menopause is a normal event in a woman's life.

In 1985 McPherson argued that nurses should collect stories of their experiences with osteoporosis and share their knowledge with other women to correct the belief promulgated in the early 1980s that osteoporosis is part of the menopause syndrome. Underlying the argument is the feminist science perspective that a dynamic health relationship exists between the investigator and the

This study was partially supported by funding from NIH, NCNR grant no. 1 R21 NU 01049; NRE/DPN grant no. NU 00455; and PHS, HRSA grant no. NR 06121.

woman. Webster, Dan, and McElmurry (1987) agreed that a collaborative relationship exists between the health care provider and a woman in which the latter can initiate or manage her own health care, with the former enhancing the client's options.

The purpose of the study from which these stories were drawn was to identify threats to sexuality in perimenopausal women and appropriate areas for developing nursing interventions. Before beginning the study, the following assumptions were made about menopause: menopause is important to women, as it marks the end of their reproductive options; the menopause brings with it physiological changes similar to those of menarche and parturition; the person most likely to know most about the experience of menopause is the woman experiencing it; and nurses who work with perimenopausal women have a storehouse of expert knowledge to tap. Based on these assumptions, specific topics were identified as relevant in studying how women managed their perimenopausal experience. These topics were coping, self-care activities, sexuality, and natural menopause. The discussion that follows offers some of the authors' goals and methods in collecting the women's and nurses' stories of menopause and presents areas for further research.

LITERATURE REVIEW

Relatively little research has been reported about how women manage their menopausal experience, which is a remarkable observation considering the prevalence and importance of the condition. Coping, according to Panzarine (1985), is an individual matter; thus, outcomes and responses may differ markedly from individual to individual. Suls and Fletcher (1985), in a meta-analysis of the coping literature, divided coping into cognitive and behavioral acts. Little research has focused on the coping activities of menopausal women. Lennon (1982) postulated that menopause is not a stressor if it occurs when expected. However, she did note that any deviation from expectation can create a crisis.

Societal context appears to be important to women in coping with menopause and may be one reason women respond in different ways to menopause. For instance, Maoz et al. (1978) related symptom frequency in menopausal women to work status and ethnicity. Flint and Garcia (1979) and Wilbush (1982) suggested that a culture's view of menopause is an important factor in coping and that women in many cultures do not report any menopausal symptoms. Uphold and Susman (1981) found an association between self-reported menopausal symptoms and marital relationships: the quality of the marriage was related to a woman's reactions to menopausal symptoms. Polit and LaRocco (1980) found that many menopausal symptoms were related to educational attainment, work status, and present health ratings. Bart (1973) hypothesized that menopausal, married women who depend on their husbands for part of their identity invest a lot of time in activities to improve their appearance.

As with coping, there are many approaches to self-care. Dean (1981) stated that self-care activities include self-diagnosis, self-treatment, self-medication, health maintenance, and disease prevention. Dean further described self-evaluation of symptoms and self-treatment as fundamental to primary health care. Woods (1985) reported that women use a lay health network to obtain relief from mental symptoms, but use professionals for other symptoms, although quite infrequently.

Nurses have collected anecdotal stories from women about their experiences of menopause and have used the information as the basis for their practice with menopausal women (McGuire & Sorley, 1978; Pearson, 1982). Much of this information consists of practical advice and can be used by many women; however, research is needed to test the clinical efficacy of this advice.

Neugarten and Kraines (1965) culled 28 menopausal symptoms from reports in the literature. Only two of them, hot flashes and excessive perspiration, have been significantly related to menopause (McKinlay & Jefferys, 1974). Two other symptoms, vaginal dryness and bone brittleness caused by loss of bone mass, are thought to be related to decreased estrogen production by middlescent women, although no direct relationship has been established. Concerns about sexuality related to menopause include loss of childbearing abilities, changes in body image (Dan & Bernhard, 1989), loss of sexual identity (Chaiphibalsardi, 1990), and sexual dysfunction caused by tissue changes in the vagina (Leiblum, Bachmann, Kemmann, Colburn, & Swartzman, 1983).

Historically, menopause has been viewed as a disease rather than a physiological process. Menopausal women have been treated with hormonal replacement therapy (HRT), first introduced by Sevringhaus in 1935 for menopausal symptoms. Wilson and Wilson (1963) considered a menopausal woman a sexless "castrate" if she did not take estrogen replacement therapy. Currently estrogen replacement therapy (ERT) is widely prescribed to prevent bone fractures associated with osteoporosis. Nevertheless, the Food and Drug Administration attaches a health warning to all estrogen preparations. Also, the media have widely publicized the dangers of estrogen preparations, dangers such as increased risk for blood clots and uterine cancer.

Korenman (1982) listed three menopausal symptoms, hot flashes, sex tissue changes (atrophy), and osteoporosis as indications for ERT. He contended that the risks of endometrial carcinoma and gallbladder disease were high when taking ERT, but added that progestin added to the ERT regimen would reduce the risk of endometrial cancer. The cycle of estrogen/progestin preparations usually results in vaginal bleeding.

Recent gynecological, neurological, obstetrical, and endocrinological texts omit reference to perimenopause. If they do discuss menopause, it is discussed under HRT and/or aging. Women from ages 45 to 65 years are ignored. Even recent texts (Wilson & Carrington, 1988; Novak, 1988; Cunningham, Mc-Donald, & Gant, 1989; DeGroot, 1989) draw on citations written during the late 1960s or early 1970s that include studies of hormonal changes in women, age range at which menopause occurs, and characteristics of menopausal women. Thus, what exists in the literature about menopause is 10 to 15 years old. Like medical research, nursing research has studied the topics of self-management, self-care in relationship to the perimenopause, or hormonal changes during menopause that indicate a physiological process. Thus, nurses need knowledge of women's experiences of perimenopause to become health providers who encourage self-care.

METHODOLOGY

Two interview guides were developed in conjunction with other researchers with expertise in women's health to explore women's self-care/coping resources for natural menopause, premenstrual syndrome (PMS), and mastectomy with regard to how these experiences threatened their sexuality. One guide was used with nurses and one was used with the women for this study. The interview guide used with nurses contained 21 items; the guide used with menopausal women contained 20 items. Most items had numerous probes to ensure elaboration about the experience of menopause and self-care/coping responses in relation to varied dysfunctions. In our perimenopausal group, 5 nurses and 15 women were interviewed using the guides. In addition, the 5 nurses and 10 of the women completed the Kearney and Fleischer's (1979) Exercise of Self-Care Agency Scale, which measures the potential for self-care. As a follow-up, 5 additional women were interviewed after completion of the initial analysis of data from the first interviews. The 5 registered nurses selected for the interviews were working in practice areas that had extensive contact with menopausal women.

The 15 women in this study were similar to the nurses in some respects: they were all from the Midwest, they were healthy (not receiving medical care at the time of the interview), and they had all signed informed consents to participate in this study. The women ranged in age from 35 to 55 years old. The median age was 43 years old. Other descriptive statistics are summarized in Table 18-1. Five of the women classified themselves as menopausal—that is, they were no longer experiencing menses and had not for 1 full year. The other 10 women identified either a menstrual-cycle variation or the experience of a hot flash as an indication that they were nearing the time of menopause.

Protocol for Selection

The women were selected for interviews after careful screening. Each was asked if she had a history of reproductive surgery such as tubal ligation, cancer, or severe debilitating disease or illness. Each woman was also asked if she had consulted a physician for any illness or disease in the past 6 months, or if she

Table 18-1   Demographic Characteristics of Perimenopausal Women Interviewed (*N* = 15)

Variable	Value	Frequency (%)
Race	Caucasian	40
	African-American	40
	Hispanic	20
Work status	Outside home	60
	Homemaker only	40
Marital status	Single	0
	Married	66
	Widowed	0
	Divorced	34
Yearly family	0–9,999	47
income	10,000–19,999	7
	20,000–29,999	33
	30,000+	13

were currently taking ERT or any form of estrogen or progestin. Women who
responded positively to any of these items were excluded from the study.

Protocol for Interview

The women and the nurses were assured that they were free to terminate participation in the study at any time. The interviews were conducted in private
without interruptions. Each interview was audiotaped and lasted approximately
1 hour. After the interview with each woman, a comprehensive health history
including a thorough menstrual history was obtained, and a vaginal smear test
for cancer of the cervix was provided as an incentive for participation in the
study.

The questionnaires were first coded separately by two researchers, then
coded together, and finally coded in a group setting by the researchers who had
used the same data collection instrument to study mastectomy and PMS. Separately, the two researchers looked at each question and coded the individual
responses for each woman. The three research teams (menopause, PMS, mastectomy) met many times as a group. As a result of this cooperative and collaborative effort, the Self-Care Responses Questionnaire (SCRQ) was developed.
The development of this instrument is discussed elsewhere (McElmurry,
Huddleston, & Chaiphibalsardi, in preparation). The Exercise of Self-Care
Agency Scale is useful for measuring the potential for self-care. The data from
the Exercise of Self-Care Agency Scale was excluded from further analysis
when it was judged an inadequate reflection of the actual self-care health behaviors or health cognitions that the women reported.

The multigroup coding provided five themes or areas for further investigation: (1) life perspectives; (2) health experiences; (3) health explanations; (4) health relationships; and (5) self-care responses.

RESULTS: WOMEN'S RESPONSES TO PERIMENOPAUSE

After further reflection about the tentative themes, the researchers organized women's experiences of menopause according to the areas of life perspectives, health experiences of menopause, health explanations, health relationships, and self-care responses.

Life Perspectives

The areas that menopausal women described that reflected their perspective toward life included general life experiences, developmental level, attitudes about life, self-definition, and self-image. Examining life perspective or outlook helped the researchers begin to understand what was happening to the women. When the menopausal women were compared with women experiencing PMS and women undergoing mastectomy, it was apparent that the menopausal women differed from the others. They had experienced a change in their life perspectives. In some way, they had transcended their culture's negative view of them. They described themselves positively and seemed to gain this "control" by understanding what was occurring around them. They conveyed a state of "integration"; they set a new path for their lives that included others, but they were more self-directed than in previous stages of their lives.

Health Experiences of Menopause

The health experiences for menopausal women included their experiences of bodily change. Nurse experts in this study described changes in women that they had observed in their practices. These include emotional lability, nervousness, depression, moodiness, lack of interest in life, and feelings of neglect. The physical changes the nurses noted were described as "whole body changes" or a general aging process and hot flashes. The sexual changes the nurses identified ranged from feeling totally unfeminine and not wanting to participate in sexual activity to an increase in sexual libido.

According to the nurses, after menopause occurs women work hard at improving their physical appearance. The women use face creams and do "extra things" to maintain a youthful appearance. Some women gain weight. Irritability during menopause was also mentioned. It was thought that the irritability ended soon after menopause. Overall, the nurses listed the visible signs of menopause as hot flashes, perspiration, and obvious emotional upsets.

Health Explanations

The health explanations of menopause were based on the women's life perspectives. Regardless of whether these explanations were in the form of myths, misconceptions based on experiences of female relatives or friends, misinformation from public or health sectors, or explanations based on "scientifically sound" information, they were the women's way of understanding what was happening to them.

When asked how the experience of menopause was for them, the women interviewees related their perceptions of menopause to what they had heard from others. If they had not discussed it with others, they seemed to lack any preconceived perception of the menopausal experience. Many of the women expressed concern about their lack of knowledge about menopause.

Most of the women did not identify changes in their menstrual cycles or menstruation as part of the menopause; they seemed to have no reference point to guide them. The women hesitated to label themselves as menopausal. This hesitancy was expressed as uncertainties about their physical condition: some thought they might be pregnant or that they merely skipped their menses. Most of the women stated they would welcome the last cycle.

The women interviewed were primarily perimenopausal. Many had experienced variation in their menstrual cycle, and only five women had completely ceased menstruating (no menses for at least 1 year). Overall, the women viewed the experiences of menopause positively. Some had ideas about what was going to happen to them; some did not. A few women had experienced what they described as mild hot flashes, but no other symptoms were identified. The women took no prescribed medications and limited their over-the-counter drug use to aspirins and vitamins. Many of the women had a "wait and see" attitude. One was "prepared for the worst" or for a negative experience. Many of the women believed that they would experience menopausal transitions similar to their mothers' or sisters' experiences.

Health Relationships

This study found that the relationships important to menopausal women depend on their life perspectives, health experiences, and self-care activities. They also depend on communication. This study also found that the women lacked a vocabulary to describe to the nurse what they were experiencing. For example, when asked, "Are you menopausal?" one women answered, "I've skipped three menstrual cycles or menstruation times this year and four last year. What does that mean?" A literal response would be to tell the women that she has skipped three menstrual cycles or three menstruation times. Beyond that, the extant knowledge of menopause limits the nurse to respond that the woman is in the early phase (which has no name) of the perimenopause, which may be evidenced by menstrual cycle changes and other related body sensations and changes that are yet to be researched.

The nurses offered their perceptions of how health professionals, including nurses, respond to menopausal women. The nurses were fearful that health professionals would treat the women stereotypically (e.g., "ah, she's going through the change." They thought the health professionals might be likely to overlook possible health problems if they assumed that the woman was merely experiencing menopause.

Self-Care Responses: Health Activities and Health Cognitions

Health-seeking activities are reflected in the actions or cognitions of the meno-pausal women. Some of the self-care responses reported were traditional activities for women, such as shopping or cleaning house, but were explained in terms of how they were used to cope with menopause. The women described a variety of self-care responses such as taking calcium tablets for osteoporosis or dyeing their hair. The women read books, dieted, ate a balanced diet, dressed well, exercised, attended school, and worked. Interestingly, all of the responses they described were activities or actions.

The nurses listed many alternative actions for the perimenopausal women; these actions including engaging in conservations with friends, reading to educate themselves, visiting a physician, talking to someone, becoming involved in some activity, or developing an interest aside from children and home.

The nurses had many suggestions for women going through menopause. One nurse indicated she would base a care plan for the menopausal women on the symptoms or problems that the women presented. The other nurses suggested that it would be helpful to provide group meetings, emotional support, active listening, friendship, and reassurances to the women that they are experiencing a physiologically normal process. The nurses advised women not to anticipate any problems, and, if they do have problems, to determine whether they are related to menopause.

SUMMARY

Perimenopausal women's self-care health behaviors and cognitions must be examined further in relation to the transitional markers of menopause and with the recognition that women need support in identifying their perimenopausal status and in identifying changes in their menstrual cycles or body sensations. Nurse researchers need to identify specific nursing interventions for human responses to menopause that would enhance women's self-care responses. The anecdotal self-care activities and coping responses reported by women for dealing with perimenopausal experiences must be clinically tested. Also, a delineation of the self-care activities that perimenopausal women use to promote and maintain health as a response to stressors would offer an interesting study.

In this study, the women and the nurses entered into a collaborative relationship with both groups as part of the research term. As a result, five major areas for further investigation were identified: (1) life perspectives; (2) health experiences; (3) health explanations; (4) health relationships; and (5) self-care responses.

REFERENCES

Allan, J. D., & Hall, B. A. (1988). Challenging the focus on technology: A critique of the medical model in a changing health care system. *ANS, 10*(3), 22–34.

Bart, P. B. (1973, September). *Pioneers, professionals, returnees, Penelopes, and Portnoy's mother.* Paper presented to the 26th Annual Conference on Aging Women: Life Span Challenges, Ann Arbor, MI.

Chaiphibalsardi, P. (1990). Self-care responses of rural Thai perimenopausal women. Unpublished doctoral dissertation, University of Illinois, Chicago, IL.

Cunningham, F. G., McDonald, P. C., & Gant, N. F. (1989). *Williams obstetrics* (18th ed.). Norwalk, CT: Appleton & Lange.

Dan, A. J., & Bernhard, L. A. (1989). Menopause and other health issues for midlife women. In S. Hunter & M. Sundel (Eds.), *Midlife myths: Coping strategies* (pp. 51–66). Newbury Park, CA: Sage.

Dean, K. (1981). Self-care responses to illness: A selected review. *Social Science Medicine, 15,* 673–687.

DeGroot, L. J. (1989). *Endocrinologywoman* (Vol. 3). Philadelphia: W. B. Saunders Co.

Flint, M. P., & Garcia, M. (1979). Culture and the climacteric. *Journal of Biosocial Science, 6* (Suppl), 197–215.

Kearney, B. Y., & Fleischer, B. J. (1979). Development of an instrument to measure exercise of self-care agency. *Research in Nursing and Health, 2,* 25–34.

Korenman, S. G. (1982). Menopausal endocrinology and management. *Archives of Internal Medicine, 142,* 1131–1136.

Leiblum, S., Bachmann, G., Kemmann, E., Colburn, D., & Swartzman, L. (1983). Vaginal atrophy in the post-menopausal women. *Journal of the American Medical Association, 249*(6), 2195–2198.

Lennon, M. C. (1982). The psychological consequences of menopause: The importance of timing of a life stage event. *Journal of Health and Social Behavior, 23,* 353–366.

Maoz, B., Antonovsky, A., Apter, A., Datan, N., Hochberg, J., & Saloman, Y. (1978). The effects of outside work on the menopausal woman. *Maturitas, 1,* 43–53.

McBride, A. B., & McBride, W. L. (1981). Theoretical underpinnings for women's health. *Women and Health, 6*(1/2), 37–55.

McElmurry, B. J., Huddleston, D., & Chaiphibalsardi, T. (in preparation). Factor Analysis of the SCRQ.

McGuire, L. S., & Sorley, A. K. (1978). Understanding and preventing the menopausal crisis. *Nursing Practitioner, 3*(4), 15–18.

McKinlay, S. M., & Jefferys, M. (1974). The menopausal syndrome. *British Journal of Preventive and Social Medicine, 28,* 108–115.

McPherson, K. D. (1985). Osteoporosis and menopause: A feminist analysis of the social construction of a syndrome. *ANS, 7*(4), 11–22.

Neugarten, B. L., & Kraines, R. J. (1965). "Menopausal symptoms" in women of various age groups. *Psychosomatic Medicine, 27,* 266–273.

Novak, E. R. (1988). *Textbook of gynecology* (10th ed.). Baltimore, MD: Williams & Wilkins.

Panzarine, S. (1985). Coping: Conceptual and methodological issues. *Advances in Nursing Science, 7*(4), 49–57.

Pearson, L. (1982). Climacteric. *American Journal of Nursing, 82*(7), 1098–1102.

Polit, D. F., & LaRocco, S. A. (1980). Social and psychological correlation of menopausal symptoms. *Psychosomatic Medicine, 42,* 335–345.

Sevringhaus, E. L. (1935). The relief of menopause symptoms by estrogenic preparations. *Journal of the American Medical Association, 104,* 624–628.

Suls, J., & Fletcher, B. (1985). The relative efficacy of avoidant and nonavoidant coping strategies: A meta-analysis. *Health Psychology, 4*(3), 249–288.

Uphold, C. R., & Susman, E. J. (1981). Self-reported climacteric symptoms: A function of the relationships between marital adjustment and childbearing stage. *Nursing Research, 30*(2), 84–88.

Voda, A. M., & Eliasson, M. (1983). Menopause: The closure of menstrual life. *Women and Health, 8*(2/3), 137–156.

Webster, D. C., Dan, A. J., & McElmurry, B. J. (1987). Self-care responses to threats to sexuality: Mastectomy, menopause, and PMS. NRE grant report: NIH, NCNR grant no. 1R 21 NU 01049.

Wilbush, J. (1982). Historical perspectives, climacteric expression and social context. *Maturitas, 4,* 195–205.

Wilson, R., & Wilson, T. (1963). The fate of nontreated postmenopausal women: A plea for the maintenance of adequate estrogen from puberty to the grave. *Journal of the American Geriatric Society, 11,* 347–362.

Wilson, J. R., & Carrington, E. R. (1988). *Obstetrics and gynecology* (8th ed). St. Louis: Mosby-Year Book.

Woods, N. F. (1985). Self-care practices among young adult married women. *Research in Nursing and Health, 8,* 227–233.

Chapter 19

An Investigation of the Nature of the Menopausal Experience: Attitude Toward Menopause, Recent Life Change, Coping Method, and Number and Frequency of Symptoms in Menopausal Women

Connie Gleim Bareford

INTRODUCTION

Menopause is an inevitable part of every woman's growth and development. As such, menopause is a normal physiological process. Within this process, however, there is considerable variation in individual response to the physiological influence of changing hormone levels. Although some women experience few or no symptoms other than cessation of menses, other women are severely debilitated by hot flashes and depression. Variables that may contribute to this variance in menopausal symptoms have been discussed in the literature.

To date, the literature about the menopausal women has focused on life events that may occur at the time of menopause (i.e., grown children leaving home) (Bart, 1972; Crawford & Hooper, 1973). An emphasis on loss—of reproductive function, of children—that has come to label this time in a women's life has resulted in a failure to systematically examine the psychological and social as well as physiological phenomena of menopause (MacPherson, 1981).

Thus the "empty nest syndrome" has become synonymous with menopause. It is this sense of loss or "emptiness" that focuses on and reinforces a negative view of menopause. To what extent does the menopausal women share this view of the menopause as a loss, and how does this influence the experience of menopausal symptoms?

According to the literature, greater recent life change, as measured by an increase in the number of recent life events—especially those life events associated with the loss of significant others—has been associated with an increase in symptoms among menopausal women and other populations; however, the role of coping with these losses has not been adequately explained (Baldree, Murphy, & Powers, 1982; Bart, 1972; Billings & Moos, 1982; Cooke & Greene, 1981; Coyne, Aldwin, & Lazarus, 1981; Crawford & Hooper, 1973; DeLongis, Coyne, Dakof, Folkman, & Lazarus, 1982; Dohrenwend & Dohrenwend, 1974; Engel, 1983; Greene, 1976; Ilfeld, 1980; Hinkle, 1974; Jaloweic & Powers, 1981; Schaefer, Coyne, & Lazarus, 1981; Suls & Mullen, 1981; Theorell, 1974). Although studies have examined the effectiveness of different coping methods in a variety of settings and populations, no single coping method has been consistently associated with decreased symptom formation in the face of stressful recent life change (Kaplan, Atkins, & Lenhard, 1982; Kolbasa, 1979, 1982; Loewenstein et al., 1981; Myers, 1982; Rosen, Terry, & Leventhal, 1982; Schaefer et al., 1981). Clearly one cannot view the physiological milestone of menopause without considering the psychological and social phenomena that accompany such an event.

Problem

The purpose of this study was to investigate the nature of the menopausal experience based on the assessment of physiological and psychosocial variables within women's lives. In this view, the influence of attitudes toward the menopause on the incidence of menopausal symptoms was investigated. Concurrent recent life change was studied to determine its role in the incidence of symptoms. In addition, the nature of a woman's coping method or manner of dealing with a stressful event was examined to determine its effect on symptom formation.

Theoretical Framework

The investigation began by asking to what extent does the menopausal woman share the view of the menopause as a loss, and how does this influence the experience of menopausal symptoms? Lazarus's framework of stress and adaptation was chosen to provide a theoretical base from which to consider the dynamics of the menopause as a multifocal event within the life cycle (Lazarus, 1980; Lazarus, Cohen, Folkman, Kanner, & Schaefer, 1980). Lazarus defines stress as a potentially damaging or challenging encounter with the environment and defines adaptation as successful coping with this encounter. The process by which stress leads to coping and adaptation involves several parts: mediating cognitive appraisal (primary and secondary), emotional response, and coping (Lazarus, 1980). Primary cognitive appraisal occurs initially as the individual perceives an event as either a loss, a threatened loss, or a challenge. According to Lazarus, attitude toward a stressful event is defined as the primary cognitive appraisal of threat (Lazarus, Averill, & Opton, 1974). Concurrent with primary cognitive appraisal are emotional changes (positive or negative). Coping is the "action" taken and is based on the entire cognitive appraisal and concurrent emotional changes, as well as feedback about the success of coping with events in the past. Adaptation is successful coping; maladaptation may be measured by the number and frequency of symptoms experienced by the individual (Lazarus, 1971).

Hypotheses and Research Question

Based on the theoretical framework and previous research, the following hypotheses were tested:

Hypothesis 1 The number and frequency of menopausal symptoms that a woman experiences is related to selected aspects of her attitude toward menopause as follows:

(1a) as negative affect increases, then the number and frequency of menopausal symptoms increases;

(1b) as psychological loss increases, then the number and frequency of menopausal symptoms increases;

(1c) as postmenopausal recovery increases, then the number and frequency of menopausal symptoms decreases.

Hypothesis 2 The number and frequency of menopausal symptoms is positively related to recent life change: Women who have experienced greater recent life change will be more likely to experience an increase in the number and frequency of menopausal symptoms.

Hypothesis 3 Attitude toward menopause and recent life change interacts with respect to the number and frequency of menopausal symptoms: The combined effect of attitude toward menopause and recent life change on the number and frequency of menopausal symptoms that a woman experiences will be greater than each considered separately.

In addition, the following research question was asked: Is a woman's coping method in response to a recent stressful event related to her attitude toward the menopause and to the number and frequency of symptoms she experiences during the menopause?

METHODS

This study employed retrospective survey techniques. Participants were recruited from various community groups and occupational settings. A sample of 103 menopausal women was identified based on self-reported menopausal status. The sample was limited to women currently undergoing menopause. In an effort to eliminate variation in hormone levels unrelated to developmental menopausal changes, women with a history of mastectomy, hysterectomy, oophorectomy, adrenalectomy, or Addison's disease, as well as women who were currently receiving estrogen replacement therapy, were excluded. Women who were experiencing interrupted menses because of pregnancy or lactation were excluded. Menopausal status was measured by a demographic survey designed by this investigator. Participants completed the questionnaires at their convenience and returned them to the author by mail.

Definition of Terms

Menopause   This refers to the actual cessation of menstruation and is said to occur after a woman has had no menstrual bleeding for at least 1 year (Dyer, 1979). Although in the United States the average age of menopause is 50 years, this event may occur with individual variation from 35 to 60 years of age (Martin, 1978).

Menopausal   This refers to women who have at some time in the past 12 months had irregularities in menstrual bleeding as compared with the previous 12 months or who ceased to menstruate within the past 12 months (Dyer, 1979).

Menopausal Symptoms   These are the commonly identified psychological and physiological complaints associated with the gradual regression of ovarian hormonal function (Uphold & Susman, 1981). Menopausal symptoms are self-reported using the Menopause Symptom Checklist (MSC) as adapted by Neugarten and Kraines (1965) from Blatt's Menopausal Index (Blatt, Weisbader, & Kupperman, 1953). Examples of menopausal symptoms are hot flashes, irritability, dizziness, headaches, tired feelings, and trouble sleeping.

Attitude   This is a learned predisposition to respond in a consistently favorable or unfavorable manner with respect to a given object (Fishbein & Ajzen, 1975). Attitude is based on an individual's perception of an object as threatening or nonthreatening (Lazarus, Averill, & Opton, 1974). Attitude toward menopause will be measured using the Attitudes-Toward-Menopause Checklist (ATM) designed by Neugarten, Wood, Kraines, and Loomis (1963). The subscales of the ATM are: (I) negative affect, (II) postmenopausal recovery, (III) psychological loss, (IV) extent of change, (V) control over symptoms, (VI) unpredictability, and (VII) sexuality. The three aspects of attitude toward the menopause that were investigated in this study are: negative affect, psychological loss, and postmenopausal recovery.

Negative Affect   (Measured by factor I on the ATM.) Using a Likert scale, respondents are asked to agree or disagree with statements describing menopause as an event that is disagreeable, depressing, troublesome, unpleasant, or disturbing.

Psychological Loss   (Measured by factor III on the ATM.) Using a Likert scale, respondents are asked to agree or disagree with statements that describe menopause as a time during which a woman's identity as a "real woman" is lost, during which a woman fears "losing her mind," and when she is concerned with how her husband will feel toward her after menopause.

Postmenopausal Recovery   (Measured by factor II on the ATM.) Using a Likert scale, respondents are asked to agree or disagree with statements describing the postmenopausal woman as feeling better, more confident, calmer, and freer than before the menopause.

Coping   Coping involves the cognitive and behavioral efforts needed to master, minimize, tolerate, or reduce internal and environmental demands and the conflict among them in stressful transactions between the person and the environment (Folkman & Lazarus, 1980; Lazarus, 1966, 1980; Lazarus & Launier, 1978).

Coping Method   This is the individual strategy used in response to a stressful life event as measured by Lazarus's Ways of Coping Checklist (WCC) (Folkman & Lazarus, 1980). Coping methods are categorized as: (1) Problem-focused methods that attempt to alter the environment in an effort to cope with stress. For example, "I try to analyze the problem to understand it better," and "I make a plan of action and follow it"; (2) Emotion-focused methods that attempt to alter one's own behavior in an effort to cope with stress. For example, "I daydream" or "look for the silver lining"; "accept it since nothing can be done"; and "try to forget the whole thing."

Recent Life Change   This involves life events for the individual that have occurred in the past 6 months and quantified in accord with Holmes and Rahe (1967) but using the 1974 revision of The Social Readjustment Rating Scale, which scores Life Change Units (LCU) based on the number of life events that are either indicative of or require some change (positive or negative) and the degree of change required for each event. For example, "death of a spouse" would add 100 points to the LCU score, whereas "a vacation" would add 13 points to the LCU score.

The dependent variable of number and frequency of menopausal symptoms was self-reported and was measured using the MSC. Independent variables were measured as follows: Attitude toward the menopause was measured using the ATM. Three aspects of attitude toward menopause were measured using three subscales of the ATM: negative affect, postmenopausal recovery, and psychological loss. Recent life change was measured by the Recent Life Change Questionnaire (RLCQ) designed by Holmes and Rahe (1967). Finally, individual strategies used in response to a recent stressful life event were measured by the WCC. Coping methods were categorized as problem-focused or emotion-focused. The instruments were presented in rotation to minimize set bias regarding the term "menopause."

Data were analyzed using a multiple regression problem for the Apple II/IIe/IIc (Regress II) (Madigan & Lawrence, 1983). Since education and employment were identified in previous research as influencing attitude toward the menopause, they were entered in a covariate design (Kresovich, 1980; LaRocca & Polit, 1980; Polit & LaRocca, 1980). Multiple regression analysis was performed to determine the best possible predictor or set of predictors of the number and frequency of menopausal symptoms and the amount of variance explained by each independent variable.

RESULTS

To check for multicollinearity, principal component analysis was performed as part of the multiple regression program. The Regress II program tests for conditions producing R-squared values greater than .99. If such a problem arises, the regression programs halt and report the condition.

Multiple regression analysis was performed entering the control variables education and employment and then all independent variables. Since education and employment made no significant contribution to the variance in number and frequency of menopausal symptoms, they were eliminated in later analyses.

Based on multiple regression analyses, the best predictors for explaining the number and frequency of menopausal symptoms is a formula containing negative affect, recent life change, and the interaction of postmenopausal recovery and recent life change, $F(1, N = 98) = 3.626$, $p = .008$ (Table 19-1).

Hypothesis 1 states that the number and frequency of menopausal symptoms that a woman experiences is related to selected aspects of her attitude toward the menopause as follows: (1a) as negative affect increases, then the number and frequency of menopausal symptoms increases; (1b) as psychological loss increases, then the number and frequency of menopausal symptoms increases; (1c) as postmenopausal recovery increases, then the number and frequency of menopausal symptoms decreases.

Hypothesis 1a was supported. Attitude toward the menopause negative affect was significantly related to an increase in the number and frequency of menopausal symptoms. Attitude toward the menopause negative affect had a unique contribution to R-square of 5.5%. Other aspects of attitude toward the menopause (postmenopausal recovery and psychological loss) did not contribute to any significant variation in number and frequency of menopausal symptoms. Hypotheses 1b and 1c were not supported.

Hypothesis 2 states that the number and frequency of menopausal symptoms is positively related to recent life change: Women who experience greater recent life change will be more likely to experience an increase in the number and frequency of menopausal symptoms than women with less recent life change.

In this study, recent life change did account for a significant portion of the variation in menopausal symptoms. Recent life change had a unique contribution to R-square of 2.2%. Hypothesis 2 was supported (Table 19-1).

Hypothesis 3 states that attitude toward menopause and recent life change interacts with respect to the number and frequency of menopausal symptoms: The combined effect of attitude toward the menopause and recent life change on the number and frequency of menopausal symptoms that a woman experiences will be greater than each considered separately.

As measured by the subscale postmenopausal recovery, a positive attitude toward menopause interacts with recent life change and is associated with a significant decrease in the number and frequency of menopausal symptoms. This interaction had a unique contribution to R-square of 3.2%. Negative attitude toward menopause as measured by negative affect or psychological loss was not enhanced by few recent life changes; there were no significant changes in the number and frequency of menopausal symptoms. Hypothesis 3 was partially supported (Table 19-1).

The research question asks: Is a woman's coping method in response to a recent stressful event related to her attitude toward menopause and to the number and frequency of symptoms she experiences during menopause? Although there were significant relationships between aspects of attitude toward menopause and the number and frequency of symptoms, there were no significant correlations between attitude toward menopause and method of coping (Table

Table 19-1   Summary of the Variance in Number and Frequency of Menopausal Symptoms[a] [F(4, N = 98) = 3.626, p = .008]

Variables	Coefficient	SE	p	$sr^{2\,b}$
ATM				
Negative affect (ATT I)	.658548	.2815	.0202	.055377
Postmenopausal recovery (ATT II)	.450596	.4167	.2818	.0104887
Recent life change (LCU)	.165703	.0741	.0259	.0224885
Interaction 2				
Postmenopausal recovery × recent life change	−.006964	.0035	.0480	.0330661

R-square = .1289; SE = 10.8422; total variance explained = 12.89%.
ATT I, negative affect; ATT II, postmenopausal recovery.
[a]Expresses the best predictors of menopausal symptoms based on a forced entry solution to the regression equation.
[b]Expresses the unique contribution of each variable as a portion of the total variance in menopausal symptoms.

Table 19-2   Zero-Order Correlation Matrix for Education, Employment, Menopausal Symptoms, Attitude Toward the Menopause, Recent Life Change, and Coping Method (n = 103).

	EDUC	EMP	SX	ATT I	ATT II	ATT III	LCU	WCCP	WCCE	WCCC
EDUC										
EMP	[b].3235									
SX	−.0397	−.1208								
ATT I	−.1177	−.1526	[a].2410							
ATT II	−.1018	−.1106	−.0615	.1280						
ATT III	−.1346	−.0573	.1270	[b].5664	[b].2553					
LCU	.1598	.0543	.1853	.1427	.0176	.1107				
WCCP	.1571	[b].2165	.0426	−.1489	.0194	.0428	.1615			
WCCE	−.0369	.1659	.1510	.0423	.0325	.1135	[b].2594	[b].6635		
WCCC	−.0278	−.0153	.1280	.1056	.0831	.1082	[b].3251	.2698	[b].4822	

EDUC, education; EMP, employment; SX, number and frequency of menopausal symptoms. Attitudes toward menopause: ATT I, negative affect; ATT II, postmenopausal recovery; ATT III, psychological loss; LCU, recent life change; WCCP, ways of coping—problem-focused coping scale; WCCE, ways of coping—emotion-focused coping scale; WCCC, ways of coping—combined coping scale.
[a]$p < .05$, two tailed .195.
[b]$p < .01$, two tailed .254.

19-2). There was no significant correlation between coping method and number and frequency of menopausal symptoms.

DISCUSSION

Based on Lazarus's theoretical framework, it was predicted that menopausal women who perceived menopause as threatening would experience an increase in the number and frequency of menopausal symptoms as compared to women who perceived menopause as a more positive event—as a challenge rather than a threat. In this study, women who perceived menopause as having a negative effect did report a significantly greater number and frequency of symptoms, whereas women who perceived menopause as a psychological loss did not report greater number and frequency of symptoms. Conversely, women who viewed menopause more positively did not report fewer symptoms.

Three aspects of attitude toward menopause were measured in an attempt to explain the variance in menopausal symptoms. Attitude was defined as a learned predisposition to respond in a consistently favorable or unfavorable manner with respect to a given object (Fishbein & Ajzen, 1975). It was assumed that the ATM subscales negative affect and psychological loss measured a negative attitude toward menopause. The subscale negative affect asked a participant to agree or disagree with statements describing menopause as an event that is disagreeable, depressing, troublesome, unpleasant, or disturbing. The subscale psychological loss asked a participant to agree or disagree with statements that describe menopause as a time during which a woman's identity as a "real woman" is lost, during which a woman fears "losing her mind," and when she is concerned with how her husband will feel toward her after menopause. A distinction may be made in comparing these two subscales as measures of negative attitude. The subscale negative affect focuses on the effects of menopause itself, whereas the subscale psychological loss assesses the part menopause plays in a woman's total development. Although both subscales may be measures of negative attitude, one needs to examine how an attitude may be learned to account for the variance in reported symptoms.

The influence of negative attitude on the incidence of symptoms has been well supported in the literature in menopausal and perimenstrual research. The unique contribution of negative affect on number and frequency of symptoms in this study is based on precedent. Woods (1985) describes the influence of negative attitude and symptoms as part of a different kind of learning process. The negative attitude may be a function of the woman's experiences with the symptoms (themselves), which are debilitating. As relates to Lazarus's framework, the cognitive appraisal of the event and concurrent emotional changes constitute feedback about successful coping. In this case, the woman complaining of symptoms is experiencing physical discomfort (i.e., feedback that coping is "unsuccessful"). She experiences a sense of failure in her ability to control these symptoms, and consequently she comes to view the event (menopause or the menses) in an unfavorable (negative) manner. Given the dynamics of negative attitude formation as previously discussed, it is difficult to speculate why positive attitude in and of itself did not account for a significant part of the variance in menopausal symptoms in this study.

Positive attitude toward menopause as measured by the postmenopausal recovery subscale of the ATM has been documented as a function of age and menopausal stage by several investigators (Dege & Gretzinger, 1982; Kresovich, 1980; Neugarten et al., 1963). In these studies menopausal and postmenopausal women were more likely to hold a positive attitude toward menopause than their younger counterparts. Perhaps one needs to distinguish the difference between the lack of a negative attitude from the possession of a positive attitude. Measurement of positive attitude was assumed to indicate agreement with the statements on the subscale postmenopausal recovery. Statements on the subscale assess a participant's agreement with the idea of a postmenopausal recovery—a positive view of the menopause, to be sure, but one that views the benefits of menopause as occurring after its completion.

An increased incidence of symptoms has been associated with recent life change in menopausal women and other populations (Bart, 1972; Billings & Moos, 1982; Cooke & Greene, 1981; Crawford & Hooper, 1973; Delongis et al., 1982; Dohrenwend & Dohrenwend, 1974; Engel, 1983; Greene, 1976; Hinkle, 1974; Jaloweic & Powers, 1981; Schaefer et al., 1981; Suls & Mullen, 1981; Theorell, 1974). The present study confirms previous research.

Specifically, an increase in recent life events has been associated with an increase in both menopausal and perimenstrual symptoms. In two recent studies, stressful life events have been associated with the onset of symptoms as part of a complex theoretical relationship. In a study of 239 women of all ages, recent stressful life events as measured by the Life Experiences Survey was directly related to perceived health status; those women who reported many recent life changes were more likely to perceive themselves as being in poor health (Engel, 1983). Negative perceived health status in turn was directly related to an increase in reported symptoms as measured by the MSC. In a study of premenopausal women, Woods (1985) measured recent life change using Holmes and Rahe's RLCQ and found that recent life change was significantly related to a negative attitude toward the menses as measured by the Moos Menstrual Inventory. An increase in negative attitude toward the menses was in turn associated with a significant increase in reported perimenstrual symptoms. In light of these findings one would expect to find a significant relationship between the interaction of recent life events and attitude toward the menopause.

The interaction between positive attitude and recent life change is well documented in the literature. Based on research studies conducted in a variety of settings and populations, a positive attitude in the face of stressful events has consistently been associated with a decrease in the incidence of symptoms and more successful coping (Kaplan et al., 1982; Kolbasa, 1979; Loewenstein et al., 1981; Myers, 1982; Rosen et al., 1982; Schaeffer et al., 1981). As measured by the ATM, a positive attitude toward menopause is reflected in looking forward to better times (i.e., a postmenopausal recovery). It seems consistent with Lazarus's theoretical framework that one would be able to cope successfully with recent life events with a positive attitude and that in the absence of recent stressful life events this positive attitude would be reinforced. In Lazarus's paradigm, feedback from a positive cognitive appraisal (a positive attitude toward the menopause) would be mediated by an essentially neutral encounter with the environment (few recent life changes) and would contribute to successful coping.

Given the significant contribution of negative attitude, as measured by negative affect, to the variance in number and frequency of symptoms in the study, why then is there no significant interaction between recent life change and negative attitude as they relate to the number and frequency of symptoms? Perhaps the theoretical relationship may help to explain this. If the symptoms may be debilitating as Woods (1985) describes, then the number and frequency of these symptoms would be unmitigated by few recent life changes, whereas a positive attitude would serve as a buffer to many recent life changes.

Additional Considerations

Participants frequently made personal comments in addition to their objective responses to the questionnaires. Personal comments of the respondents who accounted for missing data on the ATM indicated that they may have misunderstood the directions. Other participants expressed a preference to respond "no opinion" and since this was not an option they did not complete the response. Bowles (1986) states that although the ATM provides a wealth of information about a woman's attitude toward menopause, it is a lengthy instrument, and when used as part of a packet of instruments in multidimensional research, respondents are in danger of being "oversurveyed." Perhaps missing data in the present study was a consequence of the length of the survey packet.

The second most frequent source of participants' comments was related to the WCC. In this case, comments were essentially positive and offered the researcher additional data about coping methods than was measured on the WCC. Participants' comments reflected use of humor as a coping tool. One woman wrote, "Guinness Book of Records here I come . . . 40 years and I'm still menstruating! When will it ever end?" In all 66 items on the WCC none of the items mentions any use of humor. Although the checklist allows respondents to add as item 67 "any method different than the others listed," few respondents offered any alternatives. In comparison, respondents' comments reflecting the possible importance of humor as a coping tool were scattered throughout the survey packets. That the participants chose to share these comments with the researcher may indicate that humor is a relevant behavior for this particular group of respondents (Baker, 1985).

Recommendations for further research based on these additional observations would include the use of personal interviews. Within a structured format, personal interviews may address the problem of incomplete data by providing the participants with a means of clarifying directions. In an unstructured portion of a personal interview, respondents' comments regarding humor as a coping method may provide information that could be used to modify existing coping measures or to develop a new coping instrument.

Additional findings of interest concerned the types of life events reported by the respondents. The most frequently checked event of the RLCQ was listed as "a major personal achievement." Other frequently listed events were "increased responsibilities on the job," "job promotion," and "increase in income." Further analysis of this recent life change data may provide information that will serve to document this time in a woman's life as one of positive change and not loss.

SUMMARY

Three hypotheses were tested to determine the relationship between attitude toward the menopause, recent life events, and the number and frequency of symptoms in menopausal women. In addition, the research question was addressed in an attempt to determine the relationship between a menopausal woman's coping method and the number and frequency of symptoms.

Relative to the principal areas of investigation, the results of the analysis of the data revealed that a negative attitude toward the menopause—as measured by the negative affect subscale—and recent life change accounted for significant portions of the variance in number and frequency of symptoms in menopausal women in this sample. There were no statistically significant relationships between other aspects of attitude toward the menopause—as measured by postmenopausal recovery or psychological loss—and the number and frequency of menopausal symptoms. When the interactions between attitude variables and recent life change were regressed onto the number and frequency of symptoms, there was a significant inverse relationship between the interaction of a positive attitude (postmenopausal recovery) with recent life change and the number and frequency of symptoms. Multiple correlation analysis revealed that a woman's coping method did not significantly contribute to either her attitude toward menopause or variance in symptoms.

Based on the data analysis of this study, the relationship of attitude to the variance in symptoms in menopausal women is a complex one. The role of recent life change in the development of symptoms appears to be an interactive one. As a result of this study, the role of coping method in the number and frequency of symptoms requires further investigation.

REFERENCES

Baker, C. M. (1985). Maximizing mailed questionnaire responses. *Image: The Journal of Nursing Scholarship, 17,* 118–121.

Baldree, K. S., Murphy, S. P., & Powers, M. J. (1982). Stress identification and coping patterns in patients of hemodialysis. *Nursing Research, 31,* 107–112.

Bart, P. B. (1972). Depression in middle-aged women. In J. M. Bardwick (Ed.), *Readings in the psychology of women* (pp. 134–142). New York: Harper & Row.

Billings, A. C. & Moos, R. H. (1982). Stressful life events and symptoms: A longitudinal model. *Health Psychology, 1,* 99–117.

Blatt, M. H. G., Weisbader, H., & Kupperman, H. S. (1953). Vitamin E and the climacteric syndrome. *Archives of Internal Medicine, 91,* 792–799.

Bowles, C. (1986). Measure of attitude toward menopause using the semantic differential model. *Nursing Research, 35,* 81–85.

Cooke, D. J. & Greene, J. G. (1981). Types of life events in relation to symptoms at the climacterium. *Journal of Psychosomatic Research, 25*(1), 5–11.

Coyne, J. C., Aldwin, C., & Lazarus, R. S. (1981). Depression and coping in stressful episodes. *Journal of Abnormal Psychology, 90,* 439–447.

Crawford, M. P. & Hooper, D. (1973). Menopause, aging, and family. *Social Science and Medicine, 7,* 469–482.

Dege, K. & Gretzinger, J. (1982). Attitudes of families toward menopause. In A. M. Voda, M. Dinnerstein, & S. R. O'Donnell (Eds.), *Changing perspectives on menopause* (pp. 59–69). Austin: University of Texas Press.

DeLongis, A., Coyne, J. C., Dakof, G., Folkman, S., & Lazarus, R. (1982). Relationship of daily hassles, uplifts, and major life events to health status. *Health Psychology, 1,* 119–136.

Dohrenwend, B. S., & Dohrenwend, B. P. (1974). *Stressful life events: Their nature and effects.* New York: John Wiley & Sons.

Dyer, R. A. M. (1979). Menopause. In D. K. Kjernik & I. M. Martinson (Eds.), *Women in stress: A nursing perspective* (pp. 303–318). New York: Appleton-Century-Crofts.

Engel, N. S. (1983). Menopausal stage, current life change, attitude toward women's roles, and perceived health status in middle-aged women. Unpublished doctoral dissertation, New York University.

Fishbein, M., & Ajzen, I. (1975). *Belief, attitude, intention and behavior: An introduction to theory and research.* Reading, MA: Addison-Wesley.

Folkman, S., & Lazarus, R. S. (1980). An analysis of coping in a middle-aged community sample. *Journal of Health and Social Behavior, 21,* 219–239.

Greene, J. G. (1976). A factor analytic study of climacteric symptoms. *Journal of Psychosomatic Research, 20,* 425–430.

Hinkle, L. E. (1974). The effect of exposure to cultural change, social change, and changes in interpersonal relationships on health. In B. S. Dohrenwend & B. P. Dohrenwend (Eds.), *Stressful life events: Their nature and effects* (pp. 9–43). New York: John Wiley & Sons.

Holmes, T. H., & Rahe, R. H. (1967). The social readjustment rating scale. *Journal of Psychosomatic Research, 11,* 213–218.

Ilfeld, F. W. (1980). Coping styles of Chicago adults: Description. *Journal of Human Stress, 6*(2) 2–10.

Jaloweic, A., & Powers, M. J. (1981). Stress and coping in hypertensive patients and emergency room patients. *Nursing Research, 30,* 10–15.

Kaplan, R. M., Atkins, C. J., & Lenhard, L. (1982). Coping with a stressful sigmoidoscopy: Evaluation of cognitive and relaxation preparations. *Journal of Behavioral Medicine, 5*(1), 67–82.

Kolbasa, S. C. (1979). Stressful life events, personality, and health: An inquiry into hardiness. *Journal of Personality, 37,* 1–11.

Kolbasa, S. C. (1982). Commitment and coping in stress resistance among lawyers, *Journal of Personality and Social Psychology, 42,* 707–717.

Kresovich, E. A. S. (1980). A comparison of attitudes toward the menopause held by women during three phases of the climacterium. *Issues in Mental Health Nursing, 2,* 59–69.

LaRocca, S. A. & Polit, D. F. (1980). Women's knowledge about the menopause. *Nursing Research, 29,* 10–13.

Lazarus, R. S. (1966). *Psychological stress and the coping process.* New York: McGraw-Hill.

Lazarus, R. S. (1971). The concepts of stress and disease. In L. Levi (Ed.), *Society, stress and disease* (vol. 1) (pp. 53–58). London: Oxford University Press.

Lazarus, R. S. (1980). The stress and coping: A paradigm. In L. A. Bond & J. C. Rosen (Eds.), *Competence and coping during adulthood* (pp. 28–74). Hanover, NH: University of New England Press.

Lazarus, R. S. (1981). The costs and benefits of denial. In B. S. Dohrenwend & B. P. Dohrenwend (Eds.), *Stressful life events and their contexts* (pp. 131–156). New York: John Wiley & Sons.

Lazarus, R. S., Averill, J. R., & Opton, Jr., E. M. (1974). The psychology of coping: Issues of research and assessment. In G. Coelho, D. Hamburg, & J. Adams (Eds.), *Coping and adaptation* (pp. 249–315). New York: Basic Books.

Lazarus, R. S., Cohen, J. B., Folkman, S., Kanner, A., & Schaefer, C. (1980). Psychological stress and adaptation: Some unresolved issues. In H. Selye (Ed.), *Selye's Guide to Stress Research* (vol. 1) (pp. 90–117). New York: Van Nostrand Reinhold.

Lazarus, R. S., & Launier, R. (1978). Stress-related transactions between person and environment. In L. A. Pervin & M. Lewis (Eds.), *Perspectives in interactional psychology.* New York: Plenum.

Loewenstein, S. F., Bloch, N. E., Campion, J., Epstein, J. S., Gale, P., & Salvatore, M. (1981). A study of satisfaction and stresses of single women in midlife. *Sex Roles, 7,* 1127–1141.

MacPherson, K. K. (1981). Menopause as disease: The social construction of a metaphor. *Nursing Science, 3*(2), 95–113.

Madigan, S., & Lawrence, V. (1983). *Regress II: A multiple regression program for the Apple II/IIe/IIc* [Computer program manual]. Northridge, CA: Human Systems Dynamics.

Martin, L. L. (1978). *Health care of women.* New York: J. B. Lippincott.

Myers, H. F. (1982). Coping styles and competence as mediators of self-reported responses to stress. *Psychological Reports, 50,* 303–313.

Neugarten, B. & Kraines, R. (1965). "Menopausal symptoms" in women of various ages. *Psychosomatic Medicine, 27,* 266–273.

Neugarten, B., Wood, V., Kraines, R. J., & Loomis, B. (1963). Women's attitudes toward the menopause. *Vita Humana, 6,* 141–151.

Polit, D. F. & LaRocca, S. A. (1980). Social and psychological correlates of menopausal symptoms. *Psychosomatic Medicine, 42,* 332–345.

Rosen, T. J., Terry, N. S., & Leventhal, H. (1982). The role of esteem and coping in response to threat communication. *Journal of Research in Personality, 16*(1), 90–107.

Schaefer, C., Coyne, J. C., & Lazarus, R. S. (1981). The health-related functions of social support. *Journal of Behavioral Medicine, 4,* 381–406.

Suls, J. & Mullen, B. (1981). Life change and psychological distress: The role of perceived control and desirability. *Journal of Applied Social Psychology, 11,* 379–389.

Theorell, T. (1974). Life events before and after the onset of a premature myocardial infarction. In B. S. Dohrenwend & B. P. Dohrenwend (Eds.), *Stressful life events: Their nature and effects* (pp. 101–117). New York: John Wiley & Sons.

Uphold, C. P., & Susman, E. J. (1981). Self-reported climacteric symptoms as a function of the relationship between marital adjustment and childrearing stage. *Nursing Research, 30,* 84–88.

Woods, N. F. (1985). Relationship of socialization and stress to perimenstrual symptoms, disability, and menstrual attitudes. *Nursing Research, 34,* 145–149.

Chapter 20

Marital Adjustment, Life Stress, Attitudes Toward Menopause, and Menopausal Symptoms in Premenopausal, Menopausal, and Postmenopausal Women

Greer Glazer and Alice Sutton Rozman

INTRODUCTION

The menopause research literature has come under considerable criticism in recent years. Three of Voda and George's (1984) suggestions for improving menopausal research include: critical examination of instruments used to study the totality of the menopausal experience (van Keep, Utian, & Vermeulen, 1982); specificity in definition of temporal aspects of the premenopause, peri-menopause, and postmenopause; and studies designed so research on meno-pause does not continue to promote human reductionism based on the assump-tion that menopause is a disease. This study is pertinent because clear and meaningful definitions were provided, multivariate statistics were used, and instruments were critically analyzed.

In previous studies investigators failed to use standardized operational defi-nitions of temporal aspects of menopausal transition. In this study, investigators used Jaszmann, Van Lith, and Zaat's (1969) definitions, which are supported by Voda and George (1984) and Woods (1982). Use of the definitions will enable discussion of studies that address temporal aspects of menopausal symptoms. Menopause was divided into three phases: premenopausal, to describe the phase during which women have had a menstrual period within the past 3 months (less than 90 days); menopausal, to describe the phase during which menstrual periods have stopped for 3–12 months (91 days–365 days); and postmenopausal, to describe the phase during which menstrual periods have stopped for 1 or more years (greater than 366 days) (Jaszmann, Van Lith, & Zaat, 1969). These definitions were operationalized to minimize methodological error.

In existing studies, investigators failed to emphasize the totality of the menopausal experience by focusing on one or two variables and making assumptions about the whole. In this study, the investigators recognized that obtaining information about marital adjustment, life stress, attitudes toward menopause, and menopausal symptoms might appear to produce fragmentation and reductionism about menopause. However, Capra (1975) states that what makes science successful is the idea that approximations are possible. Thus, the researcher can explain many phenomena in terms of a few, and consequently understand different aspects of nature in an approximate way without having to understand everything at once. It is with this understanding that menopause was studied in terms of the four variables.

Finally, as Voda and George (1984) suggested, instrument evaluation and development is critical for a strong foundation on which to build a more holistic approach to menopausal research. The knowledge generated from this study will help to validate the usefulness of the four instruments used.

One purpose of this study was to perform psychometric testing on four instruments commonly used in studies of midlife women for determining content validity, and internal consistency and stability. This chapter relates only to this one purpose.

METHODS

Sixty-one women participated in the study. Using convenience sampling at a shopping mall and at community programs in the greater Cleveland area, researchers selected 20 premenopausal (menstrual period within the past 3 months), 13 menopausal (menstrual periods stopped for 3–12 months), and 28 postmenopausal women (menstrual periods stopped for 1 or more years). Those women with severe medical problems, with surgical or artificial menopause, or on medical treatment for gynecologic problems were excluded from the sample.

Age was not a valid indicator of belonging to a particular menopausal group. Premenopausal women ranged in age from 35 to 59 years old with a mean of 46.65; menopausal women ranged from 39 to 59 years old with a mean of 48.00; and postmenopausal women ranged from 40 to 82 years old with a mean of 61.69. This finding is particularly important because many studies have categorized women as menopausal based on age rather than menstrual status. Uphold and Susman (1981) defined climacteric women as middle-aged women between 40 and 60 years old; Cooke and Greene (1981) identified premenopausal women as being 25–34 years old; early menopausal as 35–47

Table 20-1   Selected Characteristics of Women in the Sample

Characteristics of subjects	Measure	
	Mean + SD	Range
Age in years	53.24 ± 11.26	35–82
Number of pregnancies	2.70 ± 1.98	0–9
Number of children	2.22 ± 1.52	0–8
Years of education	13.04 ± 2.80	9–26
Years together with partner	27.04 ± 11.09	1–44

years old; late menopausal as 45–54 years old; and postmenopausal as 55–64 years old. This study supports the notion that women should be classified according to menstrual status rather than age based on 40-year-old women falling into all groups. Kaufert (1986) also notes that definitions of menopausal status by self-definition, physician report, or epidemiology may not coincide. Hence, the definition of menopausal status remains controversial.

Other demographic and social data are presented in Table 20-1. The mean age was 53.24 years old; number of pregnancies 2.70; number of children 2.22; years of education 13.04; and years together with partner 27.04.

Thirty-two women were unemployed, and 27 were employed. The majority (57) of the women were white. Thirty-seven women were Catholic, 10 were Protestant, 9 were Jewish, and 6 checked "other." Thirty-eight women had a family income of over $25,000/year, whereas 23 women had a family yearly income of less than $25,000. Thirty-four (55.7%) women were married, 12 (19.7%) were widowed, 7 (11.5%) were single, 4 (6.6%) were divorced, and 2 (3.3%) were separated.

Each subject completed four questionnaires—The Dyadic Adjustment Scale (DAS) (Spanier, 1976); Life Event Questionnaire (LEQ) (Norbeck, 1984); Attitudes Toward Menopause Checklist (ATM) (Neugarten, Wood, Kraines, & Loomis, 1963); and the Menopause Symptom Checklist (MSC) (Uphold & Susman, 1981). They each also completed an information sheet. Subjects were given an identical set of instruments to complete in 1 week and return by mail for the purpose of psychometric testing.

Spanier's Dyadic Adjustment Scale

The DAS consists of 32 items that elicit subject's perceptions of the marital relationship. There are four subscales that measure dyadic cohesion, satisfaction, affection, and consensus. Each question of the scale has a fixed choice, Likert-type response of agreement or frequency, scored 0–6. Scores are added for a possible total ranging from 0 to 151. Spanier obtained content validity through the evaluation of three experts in marriage and family studies. He compared results in the same sample using the DAS and other marital adjustment scales to obtain criterion and construct validity. Correlation of results were .86 and .88 ($p < .001$). Spanier also measured reliability and obtained a Cronbach's alpha of .96 for the total scale.

Life Event Questionnaire

The LEQ (Norbeck, 1984) was used to measure life stress. The LEQ was constructed from the revision of Holmes and Rahe's (1967) original Life Change Questionnaire, the Psychiatric Epidemiology Research Interview Life Event Scale developed by Dohrenwend and Dohrenwend (1974), and Sarason, Johnson, and Siegel's (1978) Life Experiences Survey. The LEQ is a self-administered, 82-item instrument. The subject is instructed to circle whether each event that he/she has experienced in a specified time period was a "good" or "bad" event and then to indicate the amount of impact the event had on his/her life, ranging from "no effect" to "great effect" (scored 0–3). The three scores obtained are the negative events score, the positive events score, and the total events score. Test-retest correlations for adult females on the LEQ have been reported as .78 for the negative events score, .80 for the total events score, and .83 for the positive event score. The State Trait Anxiety Inventory (STAI), Profile of Mood States, and Brief Symptom Inventory were used in conjunction with the LEQ as correlates to test validity. The negative events score was the score significantly related to anxiety and negative mood states. This finding parallels Sarason et al.'s (1978) validation results.

Attitudes Toward Menopause Checklist

The ATM (Neugarten et al., 1963) is a 35-item instrument that elicits women's attitudes toward menopause. Respondents are asked to check one of the following for each statement: (1) agree strongly; (2) agree to some extent; (3) disagree somewhat; and (4) disagree strongly. Statements are worded in terms of "other women" or "women in general" rather than "self." Seven subscales were derived through factor analysis: (1) Negative Affect; (2) Post-menopausal Recovery; (3) Extent of Continuity; (4) Control of Symptoms; (5) Psychological Losses; (6) Unpredictability; and (7) Sexuality. No reports of validity or reliability were included by Neugarten et al. (1963). Bowles (1986) reported a correlation of .63 between the ATM and Menopause Attitude Scale, and a Cronbach's alpha of .80 for the ATM.

Menopause Symptom Checklist

The MSC consists of 28 of the most frequent complaints of menopausal women. Women identify symptoms they perceived during the past 12 months and whether the symptom occurred a few times or frequently. They place a mark in front of items that caused them worry or trouble in the last 12 months.

Three scores are derived from the checklist: (1) the number of symptoms; (2) severity of symptoms; and (3) Blatt menopausal symptoms. Uphold and Susman (1981) report face validity as well as test-retest correlations for number of symptoms (.79); severity of symptoms (.82); and Blatt menopausal symptoms (.70) (Kraines, 1963).

RESULTS

The aim of this study was to do psychometric testing of the four instruments (DAS, LEQ, ATM, and MSC) with premenopausal, menopausal, and post-menopausal women for the purposes of determining content validity and reliability of the instruments when used with the population of interest. Content validity of the instruments was assessed by menopause experts. Members of the Society of Menstrual Cycle Research who designated their area of interest and expertise as menopause were sent a letter by the investigators requesting their assistance in evaluating the instruments for content validity. Thirteen experts provided feedback. The following comments reflect major issues related to each instrument.

Dyadic Adjustment Scale

Two major problems with the DAS were that the scaling of items is different throughout and highly weighted on the disagree end of the continuum. Four of six options on the majority of questions are related to disagreeing. Evaluators also suggested additional items related to amount of communication, job, schooling, childbearing, health care, siblings, time spent away from partner independently, and sense of support. The DAS is useful in that it assumes neither marriage nor heterosexuality.

Life Events Questionnaire

Rating a life event as having "no effect" versus some effect confused the subjects, since they were also asked to rate the event as positive or negative. Reviewers recommended adding items such as psychologic illness, major surgery, parenting, stepchildren, taking on shared parenting responsibilities, birth of other children (either abled or disabled), having a boring job, no retirement pension, being battered by a partner, poverty, being a displaced homemaker, and having no health care insurance.

Attitudes Toward Menopause

A major problem with the ATM is the interchanging of the terms menopause and change of life. Whether these represent the same phenomenon to women is unclear. The ATM also includes items about menopause and postmenopause, thus mixing attitudes toward menopause and postmenopause. Another weakness

Table 20-2   Reliability of Instruments

	Coefficient alpha		
Instrument	Premenopausal	Menopausal	Postmenopausal
Menopause symptom checklist	.80	.81	.94
Attitudes toward menopause checklist:			
Negative affect	.86	.90	.84
Postmenopausal recovery	.83	.90	.92
Extent of continuity	.69	.49	.68
Control of symptoms	.17	.00	.01
Psychological losses	.44	.53	.66
Unpredictability	.07	.15	.26
Sexuality	.45	.44	.52
Ungrouped items	.51	.46	.32

is that the items are overwhelmingly negative. Decreasing the proportion of negative items would improve the likelihood of balanced responses to the instrument. The ATM is heterosexist, using husband rather than partner.

Menopause Symptom Checklist

Use of a symptom checklist such as the MSC is problematic for three reasons. First, it suggests things to respondents that they may not have perceived as significant, but check because the symptoms are included in the checklist. Second, whether the symptoms on the checklist are really associated with menopause is unclear. Third, the MSC places menopause within a disease model. Several of the experts believed that different responses would be elicited if women were asked to list changes or sensations they were having that were associated with menopause. Additional items suggested for inclusion on a symptom checklist included perspiration; vaginal dryness; painful intercourse; heavy menstrual flow; bleeding between periods; feeling fit, energetic, relaxed, rested; urine loss; urinary urgency; food cravings; night sweats; and leg cramps. Several experts suggested deleting flooding because of the unclarity of its meaning.

Reliability of Instruments

Internal consistency reliability was calculated for the MSC and test-retest reliability for both the MSC and the LEQ (Table 20-2). Since subscales of the ATM measure positive and negative attitudes, a total score is meaningless and reliability was only computed for the subscales. The DAS contains items with scales ranging from 2 to 7 points. Hence, inconsistency in scaling precluded reliability testing of the DAS.

Internal consistency of the instruments was determined by coefficient alpha. In genera, alpha coefficients were similar for premenopausal, menopausal, and postmenopausal women on the MSC. Reliability ranged from .80 (premenopausal) to .94 (postmenopausal) on the MSC. There was greater variation on subscales of the ATM. Alpha coefficients of the subscales of the ATM ranged from .00 ("control of symptoms," menopausal) to .96 ("negative affect," premenopausal). On the basis of the alpha coefficients obtained in this study, use of the MSC is warranted. Only two subscales of the ATM had sufficiently high alpha coefficients—"negative affect" and "postmenopausal recovery," and further use is questionable. Davis (1986) also found the ATM checklist of limited utility in her study of the meaning of menopause in a Newfoundland fishing village. The authors recommend that attitude toward menopause be measured by Bowles' (1986) Menopause Attitude Scale, which has been tested with 923 women and has excellent reliability and accepted validity.

The DAS and MSC had the highest test-retest coefficients ($r = .83$). The LEQ had a Pearson r of .48 and subscales of the ATM ranged from $-.08$ to .92. Therefore, repeated use of the LEQ and ATM is questionable from a psychometric perspective.

DISCUSSION

The greatest contribution of this study is the descriptive data that it provides and the critical analysis of instruments. Premenopausal, menopausal, and postmenopausal women were generally happily married and experiencing more positive than negative life events. As a group, women still hold negative attitudes toward menopause and experience a variety of symptoms. Use of the ATM is questionable from a psychometric perspective. Comments from experts about all four instruments raise important issues about validity, and their continued use, particularly as the only measures of a variable, is not recommended. Major implications of this study include further critical analysis of instruments before use or disuse in menopausal research, combining questionnaires with interviews to understand the context of events, and the necessity to study women on the basis of menstrual status rather than age.

REFERENCES

Bowles, C. (1986). Measure of attitude toward menopause using the semantic differential model. *Nursing Research, 35*(2), 81–85.

Capra, F. (1975). *The tao of physics.* Boulder, CO: Shambhala Publications.

Cooke, D. J. & Greene, J. G. (1981). Types of life events in relation to symptoms at climacterium. *Journal of Psychosomatic Research, 25,* 5–11.

Davis, D. L. (1986). The meaning of menopause in a Newfoundland fishing village. *Culture, Medicine, & Psychiatry, 10*(1), 73–94.

Dohrenwend, B. S. & Dohrenwend, B. P. (1974). *Stressful life events: Their nature and effects.* New York: John Wiley & Sons.

Holmes, T. H. & Rahe, R. H. (1967). The social readjustment rating scale. *Journal of Psychosomatic Research, 11,* 213–218.

Jaszmann, L., Van Lith, N. D., & Zaat, J. C. A. (1969). The perimenopausal symptom: The statistical analysis of a survey, *Medical Gynecology and Society, 4,* 268–277.

Kaufert, P. A. (1986). Menstruation and menstrual change: Women in midlife. *Health Care for Women International, 7*(1–2), 63–76.

Kraines, R. (1963). The menopause and evaluations of the self: Study of middle-aged women. Unpublished doctoral dissertation, University of Chicago, IL.

Neugarten, B., Wood, V., Kraines, R., & Loomis, B. (1963). Women's attitudes toward the menopause. *Vita Humana, 6,* 140–151.

Norbeck, J. (1984). Modification of life event questionnaires for use with female respondents. *Research in Nursing and Health, 7,* 61–71.

Sarason, I. G., Johnson, J. H., & Siegel, J. M. (1978). Assessing the impact of life changes: Development of the life experiences survey. *Journal of Consulting and Clinical Psychology, 46,* 932–946.

Spanier, G. B. (1976). Measuring dyadic adjustment: New scales for assessing the quality of marriage and similar dyads. *Journal of Marriage and the Family, 38,* 15–28.

Uphold, C. R., & Susman, E. J. (1981). Self-reported climacteric symptoms as a function of the relationship between marital adjustment and childrearing stage. *Nursing Research, 30,* 84–88.

van Keep, P. A., Utian, W. H., & Vermeulen, A. (Eds.). (1982). *The controversial climacteric.* Lancaster, England: M. T. P. Press.

Voda, A. M. & George, T. (1984). Menopause: A problem of definition. Unpublished manuscript.

Woods, N. F. (1982). Menopausal distress: A model for epidemiologic investigation. In A. M. Voda, M. Dinnerstein, & S. O'Donnell (Eds.), *Changing perspectives on menopause* (pp. 220–247). Austin: University of Texas Press.

Index